LGBTQ HEALTH RESEARCH

LGBTQ HEALTH RESEARCH

RESEARCH

Theory, Methods, Practice

Edited by
RON STALL, PHD, MPH
BRIAN DODGE, PHD
JOSÉ A. BAUERMEISTER, PHD, MPH
TONIA POTEAT, PHD, MPH
CHRIS BEYRER, MD, MPH

JOHNS HOPKINS UNIVERSITY PRESS | *Baltimore*

© 2020 Johns Hopkins University Press
All rights reserved. Published 2020
Printed in the United States of America on acid-free paper
9 8 7 6 5 4 3 2 1

Johns Hopkins University Press
2715 North Charles Street
Baltimore, Maryland 21218-4363
www.press.jhu.edu

Library of Congress Cataloging-in-Publication Data

Names: Stall, Ron, 1954– editor. | Dodge, Brian, 1973– editor. | Bauermeister,
  José A., 1980– editor. | Poteat, Tonia, editor. | Beyrer, Chris, editor.
Title: LGBTQ health research : theory, methods, practice / edited by Ron Stall,
  PhD, MPH, Brian Dodge, PhD, José A. Bauermeister, PhD, MPH, Tonia Poteat,
  PhD, MPH, and Chris Beyrer, MD, MPH.
Description: Baltimore : Johns Hopkins University Press, 2020. | Includes
  bibliographical references and index.
Identifiers: LCCN 2019057272 | ISBN 9781421438788 (paperback ; alk. paper) |
  ISBN 9781421438795 (ebook)
Subjects: MESH: Sexual and Gender Minorities | Delivery of Health Care |
  Health Services Research | Health Equity | Minority Health
Classification: LCC RA564.9.H65 | NLM WA 300.1 | DDC 362.1086/6—dc23
LC record available at https://lccn.loc.gov/2019057272

A catalog record for this book is available from the British Library.

*Special discounts are available for bulk purchases of this book. For more informa-
tion, please contact Special Sales at specialsales@press.jhu.edu.*

Johns Hopkins University Press uses environmentally friendly book materials,
including recycled text paper that is composed of at least 30 percent post-consumer
waste, whenever possible.

CONTENTS

PART 3. INTERVENTION DESIGN AND RESEARCH

COEDITORS

RON STALL, PhD, MPH, is a professor of public health at the University of Pittsburgh School of Public Health. He started work on HIV prevention research among gay men during the early 1980s. He initially focused on health disparities and studying the many intersecting psychosocial epidemics that worked to shape the spread of HIV among men who have sex with men. At the University of Pittsburgh, he created a certificate program in LGBT health research and a training program for scholars interested in LGBT health.

BRIAN DODGE, PhD, is a professor in the Department of Applied Health Science and the Center for Sexual Health Promotion at the Indiana University School of Public Health–Bloomington. He has maintained a specific research emphasis on health among diverse groups of bisexual individuals, including some of the first National Institutes of Health–funded studies focusing on bisexual men.

JOSÉ A. BAUERMEISTER, PhD, MPH, is a Penn Presidential Professor at the University of Pennsylvania. His career has focused on developing community-engaged interventions for racial/ethnic and sexual and gender minority youth using interdisciplinary approaches.

TONIA POTEAT, PhD, MPH, is an assistant professor of social medicine at the University of North Carolina, Chapel Hill (UNC) and core faculty in the UNC Center for Health Equity Research. Her research, teaching, and clinical practice focus on HIV and LGBTQ health, with particular attention to the role of stigma in driving health disparities.

CHRIS BEYRER, MD, MPH, is the Desmond M. Tutu Professor in Public Health and Human Rights at the Johns Hopkins Bloomberg

School of Public Health. He is a professor of epidemiology, international health, nursing, and medicine at Johns Hopkins. He was president of the International AIDS Society from 2014 to 2016, and he was elected to membership in the National Academy of Medicine in 2014.

OTHER CONTRIBUTORS

Kerith Conron, ScD, MPH, Blachford-Cooper Research Director and Distinguished Scholar, The Williams Institute, UCLA School of Law

Rita Dwan, MA, project manager, American Psychological Association

Stephen L. Forssell, PhD, teaching assistant professor, Professional Psychology Program, George Washington University

Peter Gamache, PhD, MPH, MBA, MLA, president, Turnaround Achievement Network

Gary W. Harper, PhD, MPH, professor, Department of Health Behavior and Health Education, University of Michigan School of Public Health

Mark L. Hatzenbuehler, PhD, associate professor, sociomedical sciences, Mailman School of Public Health, Columbia University

Colleen Hoff, PhD, director, Center for Research and Education on Gender and Sexuality, San Francisco State University

Carl Latkin, PhD, professor and vice chair, Department of Health, Behavior, and Society, Bloomberg School of Public Health, Johns Hopkins University

Ilan H. Meyer, PhD, Williams Distinguished Senior Scholar of Public Policy, The Williams Institute, UCLA School of Law

Robin Lin Miller, PhD, professor, ecological-community psychology, Michigan State University

Angulique Y. Outlaw, PhD, associate professor, Department of Family Medicine and Public Health Sciences, Division of Behavioral Sciences, Wayne State University School of Medicine

Christopher Owens, MPH, doctoral candidate, Center for Sexual Health Promotion, Indiana University–Bloomington

Erin Riley, MPH, research program manager, Center for Sexuality and Health Disparities, School of Nursing, University of Michigan

Joshua G. Rosenberger, PhD, MPH, assistant professor, biobehavioral health, Penn State College of Health and Human Development

Ayden I. Scheim, PhD, assistant professor, epidemiology and biostatistics, Dornsife School of Public Health, Drexel University

Randall Sell, ScD, professor, Department of Community Health and Prevention, Dornsife School of Public Health, Drexel University

Shauna Stahlman, PhD, MPH, Bloomberg School of Public Health, Johns Hopkins University

Rob Stephenson, MSc, PhD, professor, Department of Systems, Populations, and Leadership, School of Nursing, University of Michigan

Rachael Strecher, MPH, senior director, Storytelling Grants, Programs, and Fellowships, National Geographic

Ryan C. Tingler, MPH, research project manager, School of Nursing, University of Pennsylvania

Karin E. Tobin, PhD, MHS, associate professor, Department of Health, Behavior, and Society, Bloomberg School of Public Health, Johns Hopkins University

Ronald O. Valdiserri, professor, Department of Epidemiology, Rollins School of Public Health, Emory University

Richard J. Wolitski, PhD, independent consultant, Washington, DC; formerly director, Office of HIV/AIDS and Infectious Disease Policy, US Department of Health and Human Services

ACKNOWLEDGMENTS

This textbook represents a collaborative effort among a large and diverse group of colleagues across disciplines and institutions. As it represents the first textbook of its kind to focus on research methods in LGBTQ health, we are dedicating the effort to the memory of Dr. Judith (Judy) Bradford, a true pioneer in LGBTQ health who was one of the founding coeditors of this project. Born in Rome, Georgia, on December 17, 1943, and a fixture in the state of Virginia (including her time on the faculty of Virginia Commonwealth University), Judy sadly passed away on February 11, 2017. As co-chair of the Fenway Institute in Boston from its inception in 2001, Judy played a key role in building a framework for LGBTQ-focused research, training, and community efforts. She was the first research scientist to head a National Institute of Health (NIH)–funded population studies center focused on sexual and gender minority health, and the first to receive NIH funding to support a T32 summer institute to train the next generation of LGBTQ health researchers at Fenway. Judy was a key influencer of NIH policy as a member of the Council of the National Institute of Minority Health and Health Disparities. She had the distinction of serving on the first Institute of Medicine (IOM) panel focused on lesbian health almost 20 years ago, and then was instrumental in the IOM's landmark report on sexual and gender minority health disparities, published in 2011. She was a passionate believer in improving the health of LGBTQ communities by performing sound research and by mentoring others on how to do this research. In her later years, Judy was also critical in bringing to the fore and collaborating on new subfields of much-needed research on bisexual health and transgender health. Judy was a tireless scientist, mentor, advocate, friend, and heroine whose wisdom will be greatly missed.

We would also like to acknowledge the essential and exhaustive editorial and logistical assistance of graduate students Sophia Geffen and Matt Hopper of Johns Hopkins University Schools of Nursing and Public Health, respectively, as well as Stephanie Creasy at the University of Pittsburgh. The final product of this textbook truly would not have been possible without their time, dedication, and attention to detail.

Last, we appreciate the contributions of all authors and coauthors of this textbook.

PART 1 INTRODUCTION TO LGBTQ HEALTH RESEARCH

Queering Research

Ron Stall, Ronald O. Valdiserri, and Richard D. Wolitski

What's Queer about Health Research Methods Anyhow?

ACADEMIC DISCUSSIONS that debate the rigor of research methods used to study health are usually framed in the abstract, with specific methodological approaches held to be more or less rigorous without regard to the context in which they are applied. This view has strong scientific appeal: by having a generally agreed-upon standard about which sampling method is the strongest, which measure is the most valid, and which study design yields the most compelling results, one can evaluate the scientific literature and so form an informed opinion as to which scientific evidence is the most credible and which actions are most likely to be effective in addressing a given human problem. While this approach may be appropriate in evaluating research conducted with many populations, particular problems emerge in applying classic research methods to small and marginalized populations, such as lesbian, gay, bisexual, transgender, and queer (LGBTQ) communities. These problems prevent the application of a "one size fits all" methodological approach to investigating and mitigating the health threats faced by LGBTQ populations. To give some examples of this problem, how do we create a sampling frame for populations that often have fluid definitional qualities and for whom public records to identify members of that community are generally nonexistent and, all too often, unwelcome to many community members? Can theoretical approaches to explaining the distribution of health and illness in a population that were developed for the general population be applied without modification to marginalized populations that have life experiences far outside those of mainstream populations? Can we confidently administer standard measures to LGBTQ populations whose psychometric properties were determined through use of data drawn from general population samples? Can we adopt interventions shown to have efficacy in randomized controlled trials among general population samples and expect to see similar levels of efficacy within marginalized communities such as LGBTQ populations?

The goal of this book is to weigh these and related questions and offer guidance to scholars interested in LGBTQ health research methods. Training and further refinement in health research methods specific to LGBTQ populations will help adapt those research methods that are generally acknowledged to be those most rigorous so that they can be used to resolve health disparities among LGBTQ communities. Thus this book was not written as a training manual in generally accepted approaches to the study of health. Nor was the book written as a review of the substantive findings of the literature on LGBTQ health, nor as a clinical guide to providing health care for LGBTQ populations, as excellent work has already begun in both of these areas. Rather this textbook was written as a guide to adapting rigorous approaches, when necessary, to the study of health and health interventions among LGBTQ communities. It is an effort to provide support to those who wish to expand the evidence base on health among sexual and gender minority populations as a means to improving the health status of these communities.

Why Is This Book Needed?

It has become increasingly clear over the past 30 years that LGBTQ populations suffer many distinct health problems at rates far higher than the general population. These health disparities, some of which have reached epidemic levels, are found not only across the many different communities that constitute the larger LGBTQ world but also across the domains of infectious diseases, chronic noninfectious diseases, psychosocial health, and social pathologies such as violence victimization. It has also become abundantly clear that gauging the extent of these disparities and addressing their danger to health will require far more than simple description of their social correlates. Effective interventions are required to resolve these health threats, and, given the severity and variety of the health disparities suffered by LGBTQ populations, they demand an ambitious and varied research agenda. Indeed, given that this research agenda and the outcomes we need to see will take many decades to achieve, this charge is so enormous that it is plain that increased attention must be devoted to training new generations of scholars in LGBTQ health research. As new scholars enter the field, it is our hope that they can extend the work that has already been done to characterize known health disparities, but also to characterize additional health disparities not yet known and move toward the design and testing of preventive and therapeutic interventions that will end these epidemics. This book has been written as a first step to providing new scholars who are entering the field of LGBTQ health research with a set of tools to help them build on the initial work that has already been done to resolve health disparities in sexual and gender minority populations.

Why Not Just Use Research Methods Already Developed to Study HIV/AIDS?

Much of the initial work that has been done in the field of sexual minority health research to date has been done in response to the now decades-long HIV/AIDS epidemic among men who have sex with men (MSM). While the research in this area has led to a sea change in the extent and quality of research that existed prior to the HIV/AIDS epidemic, the research methods used to study MSM cannot be assumed to be transferable to other sexual or gender minority populations. First, the research methods that were used to study gay men in the context of the HIV/AIDS epidemic often assumed that large populations of gay men could be sampled within well-established urban communities that have existed for many decades. This same kind of residential density cannot be assumed for lesbian women, bisexual, intersex, or transgender populations. Second, if one is to take seriously the idea that social contexts matter when explaining the distribution of health and illness among populations, one cannot transfer theory and measures developed to study health among men (and, it must be said, mostly urban white men) to the study of other sexual minority populations without critical examination. Finally, HIV/AIDS is a sexually transmitted infectious disease, which again makes the transfer of research methods to the study of noninfectious diseases, psychosocial health problems, and social pathologies problematic without critical examination. For all of these reasons, it is important to critically examine the important methodological advances that were developed to study HIV/AIDS among men who have sex with men with an eye to adapting and/or specifying them for use with the study of other kinds of epidemics and other sexual and gender minority populations—and to the study of LGBTQ health concerns *unrelated to sex*, which has, again largely due to HIV, dominated much of the literature thus far.

A Note on the Meaning of Health Disparities

Health disparities are a crucial concept in public health in that they not only focus on the issue of identifying the most crucial health problems that need to be addressed within a community but also incorporate the principle of social justice. If a population bears a greater burden of disease than what might be expected in the general population, it becomes a matter of social justice to work to lower rates of disease among those disproportionately burdened. However, the definitions and consideration of how to interpret data regarding health disparities are not simple.

What Are Health Disparities? How Are They Different for LGBTQ People?

Richard J. Wolitski and Ronald O. Valdiserri

Health disparities are a form of inequality that often goes unrecognized in LGBTQ populations. These disparities are not as immediately visible or dramatic as a violent hate crime, yet they negatively affect the health of many people and can lead to disability, premature death, and increased death rates. Health disparities exist when there are measurable differences in one or more health outcomes between one group and another. These outcomes can include population-level differences in the numbers of new or existing cases of infections or diseases, physical or mental health, quality of life, longevity, or death rates.

The concept of health disparities is a basic construct that provides a foundation for much of public health, which strives to prevent disease and improve the well-being of entire communities. Understanding which populations experience more health problems, and why some groups of individuals are at greater risk, allows for interventions to be designed and implemented to improve the health of those in greatest need. By doing so, public health can improve the well-being of disproportionately affected groups and safeguard the health of all people. Documenting and understanding health disparities experienced by LGBTQ persons are the first steps to developing effective interventions that can improve health in this population. Although health disparities among LGBTQ persons have been historically understudied, there is now a substantial body of research demonstrating that LGBTQ persons are at increased risk for multiple health problems and that there is a great need for more research, health care services, and risk-reduction interventions that are specific to, and appropriate for, the needs of this population (e.g., Hatzenbuehler 2009; Mays and Cochran 2001; Meyer and Northridge 2007; Wolitski, Stall, and Valdiserri 2008).

Some disparities are biologically determined and are not considered inherently unfair or unjust. These disparities exist because of biological differences that put one group at greater risk for a health problem compared to another group. For example, disparities in breast cancer rates between cisgender women and men are due largely to biological differences. These differences are not caused by society; they are part of our physical makeup that predisposes us to specific health outcomes.

Other disparities are determined primarily by societal influences. They result from social marginalization, discrimination, and unequal access to safe and healthy living conditions, good nutrition, and health

(continued)

care that are experienced by the members of disadvantaged groups. They may also include deficiencies in the level of effort expended to conduct research, prevent, and treat health conditions that are associated with minority status. For instance, disparities in breast cancer mortality are greater for young black women than for young white women; in part these differences are due to factors such as unequal access to quality care (Gerend and Pai 2008; McCarthy, Yang, and Armstrong 2015).

Socially driven disparities are inherently unjust and should not be tolerated (Whitehead 1992). Some authors use the term *health inequities* to distinguish avoidable disparities that result from unjust social circumstances from those that are purely biologically determined. Braveman and Gruskin (1992) describe health inequities as those that "systematically put groups of people who are already socially disadvantaged (for example, by virtue of being poor, female, and/or members of disenfranchised racial, ethic, or religious groups) at further disadvantage with respect to their health." These same constructs can, and should, include sexual and gender minorities.

Sexual and gender minorities have experienced many forms of social and legal disadvantage, yet prior to the late 1990s, sexual orientation and gender identity were often not addressed as part of research on health disparities or programs designed to reduce disparities. LGBTQ persons were often invisible in research that sought to measure health disparities because surveys did not include questions about sexual orientation or gender identity. Because the data did not exist, the number and severity of health disparities affecting gender and sexual minorities were not clearly recognized—or understood—and few public health programs (other than those related to HIV and other sexually transmitted infections) were implemented to addresses these disparities.

A number of factors might have played a role in explaining why so little attention was paid in the past to health disparities affecting LGBTQ people, including the historical invisibility of sexual and gender minorities; disregard because of the relatively small size of these populations; an exclusive focus on sexually transmitted infections that neglected other important health issues; negative societal attitudes toward homosexuality that might have caused some to ignore gender and sexual minorities or to believe that people who "chose" to be gay, lesbian, bisexual or transgender "got what they deserved." While these negative attitudes have substantially improved since the early 2000s, they have resulted in lasting gaps in our understanding and response to a wide range of health problems that have a great impact on the health of gender and sexual minorities in the United States and around the world. The gaps in our knowledge and public health response are especially great with regard to issues other than HIV that affect LGBTQ health.

Although attitudes are improving, sexual and gender minorities continue to experience institutional, social, and interpersonal discrimination that negatively affect physical and mental health. For any minority group, stigma and discrimination can affect health directly (for example, increased risk of depression, anxiety, suicide, and violence) or affect health indirectly through a number of channels, such as employment discrimination, poverty, poorer access to health care, and receipt of inappropriate or inadequate health care (Brunner 1997; King & Williams 1995; Meyer 2003; Raphael 2003; Williams, Neighbors, and Jackson 2003). However, the experiences of sexual and gender minorities have unique aspects. Sexual and gender minorities who are also racial or ethnic minorities may experience negative health outcomes related to simultaneous multiple minority status in which they experience racial/ethnic discrimination in LGBTQ communities and also anti-LGBTQ stigma and discrimination within their own racial/ethnic communities and families (McConnell et al. 2018).

Racial and ethnic minorities are typically recognized, at birth, as belonging to a minority group. They are affected by the experiences of their family members early in life, which may include the effects of stigma and discrimination, such as wealth inequality, housing inequality, and limited health care access. Gonsiorek (1995) describes racial and ethnic identities as being "vertically integrated" and sexual and gender minority identities as being "horizontally integrated." In vertically integrated groups, information and norms are passed through families from one generation to the next. For example, the effects of discrimination, unequal socioeconomic status, and health disparities experienced by earlier generations of racial/ethnic minorities can be passed on to later generations and can begin affecting health status even before birth (Gonsiorek 1995). Likewise, survival strategies for coping with stigma and discrimination can also be passed on.

In horizontally integrated groups, such as LGBTQ populations, the learning of cultural norms and information related to sexual orientation and gender identity occurs largely from peers, not one's family of origin. Because sexual and gender minority status is not related to the social circumstances into which one is born, sexual and gender minorities may begin life in more or less advantaged positions based on other factors such as race and socioeconomic status.

The chronology of sexual and gender minority identity acquisition is different from racial/ethnic minority identity acquisition. While racial

(continued)

and ethnic minority identities are generally ascribed at birth, sexual and gender minority identities are often acquired later in life, typically during adolescence or young adulthood. This chronology has important implications. The early disadvantages often associated with racial or ethnic minority group status may not be experienced by sexual and gender minorities who are not racial or ethnic minorities until later in childhood or early adulthood. Thus, all other things being equal, access to high-quality nutrition, medical care, and education during childhood is unlikely to differ for most sexual and gender minorities compared with their peers of the same socioeconomic status. It is important to recognize, however, that some children are gender nonconforming at an early age or develop traits that are associated with sexual minority status and experience discrimination early in life. Furthermore, sexual orientation and gender identity can change over time, and thus some individuals may move in and out of minority status based on their current sexual orientation and/or gender identity or presentation.

Although many sexual and gender minorities may start out life on an equal footing compared with their cisgender heterosexual peers of the same race or ethnicity and socioeconomic status, they risk losing this status as they (and others) become aware of their attraction to same-gender partners or identification with a gender other than the one assigned at birth. The process of acknowledging, acting on, and disclosing one's same-gender sexual attraction ("coming out") or transgender identity can be very stressful for many individuals. Part of this stress is associated with acquisition of a new or additional minority status and the potential losses that come with it, such as disruption of existing relationships and loss of social status and support from friends and family members (D'Augelli and Hershberger 1993; Damien and Hetrick 1988; Hetrick and Damien 1987; Strommen 1989). Thus, when sexual and gender minorities fully acknowledge their identities, they risk losing important sources of social, emotional, and financial support that can help buffer the effects of stigma, discrimination, and other stressors. This includes being rejected by one's own family, close friends, faith community, and other societal organizations. Racial/ethnic minority sexual and gender minorities risk loss of social support that helped to mitigate the negative effects of racial discrimination. Rejection by one's own family can be especially damaging for young people. Sexual and gender minority youth experience much higher rates of homelessness compared with other youth (Cochran, Stewart, Ginzler, and Cauce 2002; Moskowitz, Stein and Lightfoot 2013; Rice 2013), and a negative reaction by one's family and victimization in school have been associated with a significantly greater risk of depression, substance use, suicide, high-risk behavior, and HIV infection in adulthood (Bouris, Guilamo-Ramos, Pickard, Shiu, Loosier, Dittus, Gloppen, and Waldmiller 2010; Russell, Ryan, Toomey, Diaz, and Sanchez 2011; Ryan, Huebner, Diaz, and Sanchez 2009).

While racial and ethnic identities are often readily perceived by others, a distinct aspect of sexual and gender minority status is the potential to keep one's sexual orientation and gender identity a secret. Sexual and gender minority status is often not apparent unless it is disclosed to others, and it can be denied if it is questioned. This allows sexual and gender minorities to selectively disclose in some settings and to certain individuals, but not others. This can have beneficial effects in some settings (e.g., avoiding discrimination) but can add to the stress of being a sexual or gender minority. Keeping secrets, including hiding one's sexual orientation or gender identity, has been shown to negatively affect health (Cole, Kemeny, and Taylor 1997; Cole, Kemeny, Taylor, and Visscher 1996; Russell, Toomey, Ryan, and Diaz 2014; Ullrich, Lutgendorf, and Stapleton 2003).

The stigma and discrimination experienced on the basis of sexual and gender minority status has much in common with that experienced on the basis of membership in other minority groups, but it also has unique features. Policymakers, health care providers, educators and education institutions, public health agencies, families, and society all have a responsibility for working to eliminate stigma and discrimination and creating environments and policies that support the health of people of any sex, gender identity, race, ethnicity, national origin, religion, disability, or sexual orientation.

Adapted from R. J. Wolitski, R. O. Valdiserri, and R. Stall. Health disparities affecting gay, bisexual, and other men who have sex with men: An introduction. In R. J. Wolitski, R. O. Valdiserri, and R. Stall, eds., *Unequal Opportunity: Health Disparities Affecting Gay and Bisexual Men in the United States*, 3–32. New York: Oxford University Press, 2008.

A Note on Language to Refer to Sexual and Gender Minority Populations

We live in an era that is rich—and becoming richer—in phrases to describe LGBTQ people and communities (Bostwick et al. 2019). This complexity can sometimes lead to misunderstandings of the meaning of scientific data about sexual and gender minority populations. A division generally recognized in industrialized countries is that between terminologies that refer to behaviors (*women who have sex with women* or *women who have sex with women and men*) and those that refer to identities (*lesbian women* or *bisexual women*). Similarly, many terms exist to describe gender minority populations. For example, *intersex* describes those born with sexual or reproductive anatomy that does not align with typical cultural expectations of male and female sexual organs, while *transgender* is a commonly used umbrella term to describe a broad range of individuals whose gender identity or gender expression differs from cultural expectations based on the sex to which they were assigned at birth. These terms vary over space and across cultures. Across the global cultural record it is possible to encounter categories for sexual minority people who do not fit neatly into the categories generally recognized in the scientific literature from the global north. These categories expand even further when considered over time, as new terms to describe LGBTQ populations are constantly being coined (e.g., the use of the phrase *GMT populations* as a category to describe gay men, men who have sex with men, and transgender populations).

It is neither possible nor desirable to resolve all of this remarkable complexity, and this textbook does not offer a single taxonomy that will give readers a simple cheat sheet to interpret what any one paper or author means by a given term. We caution readers to carefully determine how specific authors are using language to describe behaviors, identities, attraction or other markers of sexual minority status as they interpret the meaning of specific chapters. Fortunately, it is often a straightforward task to sort out how these terms are being used—but care should always be taken to ensure that one is not misinterpreting the analytical categories that authors are using to describe sexual minority populations.

In this book we have settled on the use of *LGBTQ populations*. We want to be as inclusive as possible as we provide tools to bolster readers' capacities to conduct and interpret LGBTQ health research, while also acknowledging the current limitations of the science. For reasons we discuss throughout the book, methodological challenges exist in varying degrees across the various subpopulations that constitute LGBTQ communities, but we hope this book will serve as a useful resource to empower you, the next generation of scholars pursing this research agenda, to fill these gaps and move the discipline forward.

The Challenges of Language

Terminology around sexual orientation and gender identity has evolved over time and will continue to do so into the foreseeable future. These changes in language represent exciting new ways that sexual and gender minorities continue to understand and define their identities. These changes also present challenges when writing a textbook that seeks to be appropriate for a broad audience and relevant for future users. For example, many older sexual and gender minorities remember when the word *queer* was used as a pejorative term and often associated with violence in games such as "smear the queer." On the other hand, many younger sexual and gender minorities embrace *queer* as a broad umbrella term that resonates with their experience of resisting sexual and gender norms. Similarly, the term *transgender* is not universally embraced by gender minority persons. Some prefer an identity of *man* or *woman* that is inclusive of cisgender and transgender people. A growing number of gender-diverse young people identify outside of the gender binary and often use terms such as *nonbinary* or *agender* instead of *transgender*. Thus, our challenge was to select language that is respectful of the diversity of sexual and gender minority groups yet easily understandable by readers who may not be familiar with these concepts.

Throughout the text you will notice that various terms, such as LGBT, LGBTQ, LGBTQ+, sexual and gender minorities (SGM), transgender, and gender diverse, are used to describe the spectrum of gender and sexual orientation. While this may seem inconsistent at first, we feel it reflects the diversity within communities and allows the authors of each chapter the freedom to write about groups with which they are most familiar. We also acknowledge that there are language issues this book is not able to address. For example, many case studies and examples used in this book refer to "men who have sex with men," or MSM. Most of these refer to cisgender men who have sex with other cisgender men. Resisting cis-normativity requires that we be explicit about whether our terms refer to cisgender, transgender, and/or gender nonbinary individuals. Thus, our case

(continued)

studies and examples would refer to CMSCM (cisgender men who have sex with cisgender men) or CMSTM or TMSCM or a variety of other configurations that make gender visible, rather than assumed. However, the literature upon which we rely for these data simply does not provide this information. Therefore, we describe the examples and case studies as they were originally reported and call on future research to provide greater clarity.

How Is This Book Organized?

We organized this book around the idea that fields of research often develop around "generational" themes of research, each with their own specific foci and requisite skill sets. The first generation of research is that of description, during which a health disparity is first discovered to exist and is first characterized in terms of its social and behavioral epidemiology as well as its etiology and pathogenesis in clinical terms. The second generation of research is that of understanding the associations and underlying reasons for the health disparity, with the view of constructing an evidence base upon which intervention outcome trials might be attempted. The third generation of research is that of intervention research, during which the efficacy of an intervention is tested as a possible means of resolving an epidemic. The final, fourth generation of research is that of public health practice, during which the actual effectiveness of the intervention as fielded in real-world settings is evaluated.

Readers will find that we organized the book in a generations framework as a heuristic to arrange the many different methodological skill sets important to the study of health issues among LGBTQ populations. To give some examples, definitional issues are emphasized in the first part, theoretical issues in the second, and some real-life examples of intervention design in the third.

We hope that readers will also take note that the skill sets emphasized in each part build logically upon one another toward a culmination in public health practice. That is, one cannot design and test interventions for LGBTQ populations without first considering the definitional issues of who should be included in the sampling frame (generation one) or the theoretical approach that underlies the intervention (generation two). Thus, while readers who are interested in, say, intervention design might want to focus on the section that highlights third-generation research, it is important to review the chapters that lead to that discussion to ensure that important skill sets are not ignored. Similarly, those researchers who are interested in identifying the driving forces and reasons for a health disparity in LGBTQ populations (generation two) might also want to familiarize themselves with the discussion of intervention design as a way of ensuring that their work will become a crucial foundation for colleagues who wish extend their work to construct and test interventions designed to end health disparities.

How Should the Book Be Used?

The genesis of this book was a series of organized sessions on the state of training programs in LGBTQ health research at ongoing annual meetings of the American Public Health Association (APHA). During these well-attended sessions, three themes stood out in the discussions: (1) there is a great deal of interest in how best to train the next generation of scholars in LGBTQ health research; (2) while there is a great deal of interest in training issues, only a few institutions around the United States have the requisite number of faculty with experience in conducting LGBTQ health research; and, (3) while there are great numbers of students who wish to be trained in LGBTQ health research methods, few have the resources or desire to move across the United States to matriculate at programs that are fortunate enough to have the resources to support an independent training program in LGBTQ health research. In fact, the dominant picture that emerged from the APHA sessions on training in LGBTQ health research was that most schools of public health have resident students who have expressed interest in leveraging their public health educations as a means of addressing LGBTQ health disparities. As a group, we assume that the training situation in most low- and middle-income countries was even more challenging than that found among schools of public health in the United States. Thus, if we are to support the training needs of the next generation of scholars in LGBTQ health research, we need to create training platforms that go beyond traditional flagship programs in a set of well-positioned universities. The discussions that we held in response to these meetings led us to consider the possibility of creating a textbook and a set of associated online lectures to support the training needs of early-stage scholars in the field.

Given the lessons that we drew from the APHA meetings, we chose to structure the book to meet the needs of scholars who are seeking to further their educations in institutions where support of full-fledged training programs in LGBTQ health research methods is currently not possible. Hence we organized the book around the acquisition of specific methodological skill sets that are crucial to conducting research with sexual and gender minorities. We also decided that if the book was to function as needed in settings where programs in LGBTQ health research cannot be supported, the book needed to be accompanied by a set of lectures given by experts in the field, and that these lectures should be accompanied by a set of supportive readings that are available on line. Our goal was to create a combined textbook and online educational training program in LGBTQ health research that gives readers basic methodological skill sets necessary to contributing to the knowledge base in the field.

Different types of readers are likely to want to use this book in different ways. If you are among a group of students in an educational institution that cannot support a training program in LGBTQ health research, we recommend that your group organize a reading class that would use this book and the accompanying lectures as basic resources for the class. We recommend that you invite a professor or lecturer in your school to lead the class, to ensure that participation in the class is steady and that discussions of the materials remain rigorous. If you are a professor who has been asked to lead this class, we recommend that you review the materials that we selected, but strongly recommend that you add or subtract from the list of suggested readings and topics to emphasize areas where you think that the book could be improved. We are certain that with the fast growth of research in this field, new and essential readings will soon appear that would have been highlighted in the textbook had we been aware of these papers; we strongly recommend that these readings be used to expand the value of the book. If you are in a school that has a well-established training program in LGBTQ health, we hope that the book can be used as one of the training resources available at your institution. Finally, we also suspect that this book will find an audience, particularly in low- and middle-income country settings, where it may be difficult to find an instructor for a reading class. In such settings, we recommend that students come together for weekly meetings after having viewed the lectures and read the readings and relevant sections of the book, and discuss how the techniques proposed in this book might further research in your geographical and substantive areas. We strongly suspect that these discussions, and especially those conducted in low- and middle-income country settings, will be fascinating and wish that everyone who reads this book could listen and learn from these debates.

Why Was the Book Not Written with a Consistent Voice?

Because it was not written by a single person: this book was written as a collaborative effort by many different leaders in the field.

Given the range of topics that a book of this nature required, we decided to invite contributions from many of the leaders in the field of LGBTQ health research to author chapters that highlighted their expertise. Given the fact that these scientists have been leaders in the field in their areas, we thought it best to ensure that their own voices were evident in the writing and in the online lectures. To "smooth" out variations in language and in presentation style would, we believed, only produce a book that was more consistent, not one that was more valuable or more interesting. We also agreed that having variation in the way that topics are addressed would make this textbook closer to the original intent of the book: to provide an alternative to a well-resourced training program in LGBTQ health, in which students would have the experience of getting to know leaders in the field in person.

We also wanted to ensure that variation in voices is experienced by readers of this textbook in a different sense. One of remarkable and most valuable qualities of the LGBTQ social world is our diversity. It is a rare culture, indeed, in which affiliation by such a broad range of social identities is not only possible, but is affirmed, at least on our community's best days. Where this affirmation falls short is when more marginalized members of our community are not allowed a voice or when their message is devalued. We have tried, probably imperfectly, to address this gap in the research literature by inviting the participation of a broad range of scholars who identify with a diversity of gender, racial, sexual, national, and age categories. We have invited them to give commentary and write sections throughout this book, and we hope that our attempt to support diversity not only of research, but also among researchers themselves, enhances the quality of this textbook.

In closing, it should also be mentioned that the lectures and texts in this book were all provided by the authors as a volunteer effort, with no remuneration offered nor asked for by any of the contributors. None of the authors will be given royalties from book sales: rather, we hope that if there are any such royalties, they can be used to fund updates of the online lectures. That this book was produced during a time of scarce funding resources, when many of the authors were struggling to find support to continue their research efforts, is a remarkable testament to the commitment of these scientists to the support of training efforts in the field. Although not generally recognized, scientists can also be activists, too, although their style of activism is often so quiet that it goes unnoticed. That said, when scientists somehow find the time to contribute to the training of new generations of researchers in LGBTQ health research in an adverse professional environment, we hope that readers will agree that this is an effective form of activism, indeed. We hope that readers find the contributions of the authors of this textbook to be of value as they develop their own programs of research in LGBTQ health research.

Measuring Intersectional Stigma

Ayden I. Scheim

Rooting her terminology in Black feminist scholarship challenging the presumed additivity of oppressions (e.g., Collins 1990; Combahee River Collective 1979; King 1988), Crenshaw (1989) coined the word *intersectionality* to describe the discrimination experiences of Black women, which were made unintelligible by legal approaches that considered race and sex separately. Intersectionality has become a central framework for understanding multiple, interacting, and context-dependent forms of social and health (dis)advantage based on social identity and position (Bowleg 2012). McCall (2005) provides a typology of intersectionality frameworks, including the *intracategorical* and *intercategorical* approaches that have been applied to quantitative LGBT health research. These approaches share the perspective that while social categories are constructed, they nevertheless reflect real differences in power. Intracategorical studies focus on experiences at specific, marginalized intersections of social categories, while intercategorical studies examine relationships of inequality across intersections.

Discussions of intersectionality often center on identity; however, identities serve as markers of health-determining processes, including stigma being anticipated, internalized, and experienced at the interpersonal, community, and structural levels. Recognizing this, LGBT health researchers are increasingly interested in measuring exposure to stigma and its consequences from an intersectional perspective. For researchers in the nascent field of quantitative intersectionality, selecting intersectional stigma measures and analyzing the resulting data can prove challenging. Measurement decisions should be driven by theory, analytic planning, and feasibility. Below I outline measurement approaches and considerations for intra- and intercategorical studies, respectively. I focus on self-reported interpersonal stigma, as most intersectional stigma measurement takes place at this level, but note that intersectional structural stigma represents an important area for methodological development (Pachankis et al. 2017).

Intracategorical Intersectionality Studies

Intracategorical intersectional stigma measures focus on the qualitatively unique ways in which stigma manifests at specific intersections. By design, these measures tap constructs that only have meaning at particular intersections and assume shared positionality (e.g., microaggressions among LGBT people of color; Balsam et al. 2011). Alternatively, some intracategorical studies administer separate instruments for each stigma (e.g., HIV-related, gender, and racial discrimination among Black women living with HIV; Logie et al. 2013). These approaches are not conceptually equivalent, underscoring the need for careful theorizing. Arguments consistent with intersectionality can be marshalled for the use of either combined or separate

(continued)

measures. For example, gendered racism is a qualitatively unique phenomenon irreducible to the sum of racism and gender discrimination (Lewis and Neville 2015). On the other hand, one may hypothesize that racism and gender discrimination interact to produce poorer health (Marcellin et al. 2013). The extent to which intersectional stigma is qualitatively unique may depend on the level of stigma (e.g., major discrimination versus microaggressions; Sue 2010). Pragmatics and cognitive burden should also be considered; multiple measures increase participant burden and preclude valid assessment of total discrimination burden. Moreover, qualitative research suggests that multiply marginalized individuals may be unable to identify the basis of any given act of enacted stigma, raising questions as to the validity of survey measures that require them to do so (Bowleg 2008).

Intercategorical Intersectionality Studies

Intercategorical intersectionality studies require stigma measures that can be administered across intersections and that reflect shared constructs. A popular approach has been to adapt measures that were developed to assess ethnoracial discrimination but that do not specify ethnoracial identity in the question stem, such as the Everyday and Major Discrimination scales by Williams et al. (1997). Because the scales first measure exposure to "unfair treatment" and then ask for attributions to discrimination, they can be used to compute total discrimination frequency and to model the number or type of attribution(s) reported. However, because attributions are not tied to frequencies, analytic options are restricted (e.g., to counting the number of attributions reported). In addition, these measures were originally intended to ascertain anti-Black racism, and their content validity for other groups (Shariff-Marco et al. 2009) has been questioned. Bauer and Scheim (2019a) recently proposed attribution-free intercategorical measures of discrimination "because of who you are" to be used in analyses structured around intersectional social categories. Their Intersectional Discrimination Index was designed to facilitate investigations of enacted stigma as a mediator of intersectional health disparities (Bauer and Scheim 2019a).

Future Directions

Research describing the patterning of health outcomes across intersectional groups is a necessary first step to addressing health disparities faced by intersectional LGBT populations. To intervene on intersectional health disparities, it is critical that we understand their driving mechanisms. A growing number of intersectional measures of stigma and discrimination at multiple social-ecological levels enable LGBT health researchers to do so. However, as intersectionality frameworks move into quantitative health research, their complexity and methodologic implications are sometimes underappreciated (Bauer and Scheim 2019b). When designing studies to understand the health effects of intersectional stigmas, researchers should familiarize themselves with the rich theoretical literature on intersectionality and consider how they wish to analyze the data they collect. Intersectional stigma measurement remains an area of active scientific development, and opportunities abound for researchers to contribute to advancing the field.

References

Balsam, K. F., Molina, Y., Beadnell, B., Simoni, J., and Walters K. 2011. Measuring multiple minority stress: The LGBT People of Color Microaggressions Scale. *Cultural Diversity and Ethnic Minority Psychology* 17(2): 163–74.

Bauer, G. R., and Scheim, A. I. 2019a. Methods for analytic intercategorical intersectionality in quantitative research: Discrimination as a mediator of health inequalities. *Social Science and Medicine* 226(C): 236–45.

Bauer, G. R., and Scheim, A. I. 2019b. Advancing quantitative intersectionality research methods: Intracategorical and intercategorical approaches to shared and differential constructs. *Social Science and Medicine* 226: 260–62.

Bostwick, W., and Dodge, B. 2019. Introduction to the special section on bisexual health: Can you see us now? *Archives of Sexual Behavior* 48(1): 79–87.

Bouris, A., Guilamo-Ramos, V., Pickard, A., Shiu, C., Loosier, P. S., Dittus, P., Gloppen, K., and Waldmiller, J. M. 2010. A systematic review of parental influences on the health and well-being of lesbian, gay, and bisexual youth: Time for a new public health research and practice agenda. *Journal of Primary Prevention* 31(5–6): 273–309.

Bowleg, L. 2012. The problem with the phrase *women and minorities*: Intersectionality–An important theoretical framework for public health. *American Journal of Public Health* 102(7): 1267–73.

Brunner, E. J. 1997. Stress and the biology of inequality. *British Medical Journal* 314(7092): 1472–76.

Cochran, B. N., Stewart, A. J., Ginzler, J. A., and Cauce, A. M. 2002. Challenges faced by homeless sexual minorities: Comparison of gay, lesbian, bisexual, and transgender homeless adolescents with their heterosexual counterparts. *American Journal of Public Health* 92(5): 773–77.

Cole, S. W., Kemeny, M. E., Taylor, S. E., and Visscher, B. R. 1996. Elevated physical health risk among gay men who conceal their homosexual identity. *Health Psychology* 15(4): 243–51.

Cole, S. W., Kemeny, M. E., Taylor, S. E., Visscher, B. R., and Fahey, J. L. 1996. Accelerated course of human immunodeficiency virus infection in gay men who conceal their homosexual identity. *Psychosomatic Medicine* 58(3): 219–31.

Collins, P. H. 1990. *Black Feminist Thought*. Boston: Hyman.

Combahee River Collective. 1979. A Black feminist statement. In Z. R. Eisenstein, ed., *Capitalist Patriarchy and the Case for Socialist Feminism*, 362–72. New York: Monthly Review.

Crenshaw, K. 1989. Demarginalizing the intersection of race and sex: A Black feminist critique of antidiscrimination doctrine, feminist theory and antiracist politics. *University of Chicago Legal Forum* 1989: 139–67.

D'Augelli, A. R., and Hershberger, S. L. 1993. Lesbian, gay, and bisexual youth in community settings: Personal challenges and mental health problems. *American Journal of Community Psychology* 21(4): 421–48.

Damien, M. A., and Hetrick, E. S. 1988. The stigmatization of the gay and lesbian adolescent. *Journal of Homosexuality* 15(1–2): 163–83.

Gerend, M. A., and Pai, M. 2008. Social determinants of black-white disparities in breast cancer mortality: A review. *Cancer Epidemiology, Biomarkers and Prevention* 17(11): 2913–23.

Gonsiorek, J. C. 1995. Gay male identities: Concepts and issues. In A. R. D'Augelli and C. J. Patterson, eds. *Lesbian, Gay, and Bisexual Identities over the Lifespan*, 24–47. New York: Oxford University Press.

Hatzenbuehler, M. L. 2009. How does sexual minority stigma "get under the skin"? *Psychological Bulletin* 135(5): 707–30.

Hetrick, E. S., and Damien, M. A. 1987. Developmental issues and their resolution for gay and lesbian adolescents. *Journal of Homosexuality* 14(1–2): 25–43.

King, D. K. 1988. Multiple jeopardy, multiple consciousness: The context of a Black feminist ideology. *Signs* 14(1): 42–72.

King, G., and Williams, D. R. 1995. Race and health: A multidimensional approach to African-American health. In B. C. Amick, S. Levine, A. R. Tarlov, and D. C. Walsh, eds., *Society and Health*, 93–130. New York: Oxford University Press.

Lewis J. A. and Neville, H. A. 2015. Construction and initial validation of the Gendered Racial Microaggressions Scale for Black women. *Journal of Counseling Psychology* 62(2): 289–302.

Logie, C., James, L., Tharao, W., and Loutfy, M. 2013. Associations between HIV-related stigma, racial discrimination, gender discrimination, and depression among HIV-positive African, Caribbean, and black women in Ontario, Canada. *AIDS Patient Care and STDs* 27(2): 114–122.

Marcellin, R. L., Bauer G. R., and Scheim, A. I. 2013. Intersecting impacts of transphobia and racism on HIV risk among trans persons of colour in Ontario, Canada. *Ethnicity and Inequalities in Health and Social Care* 6(4): 97–107.

Mays, V. M., and Cochran, S. D. 2001. Mental health correlates of perceived discrimination among lesbian, gay, and bisexual adults in the United States. *American Journal of Public Health* 91(11): 1869–76.

McCall, L. 2005. The complexity of intersectionality. *Signs* 30(3): 1771–1800.

McCarthy, A. M., Yang, J., and Armstrong, K. 2015. Increasing disparities in breast cancer mortality from 1979 to 2010 for US black women aged 20 to 49 years. *American Journal of Public Health* 105 (Supp 3): S446–S448.

McConnell, E. A., Janulis, P., Phillips, I. I., Truong, R., and Birkett, M. 2018. Multiple minority stress and LGBT community resilience among sexual minority men. *Psychology of Sexual Orientation and Gender Diversity* 5(1): 1–12.

Meyer, I. H. 2003. Prejudice, social stress, and mental health in lesbian, gay, and bisexual populations: Conceptual issues and research evidence. *Psychological Bulletin* 129(5): 674–97.

Meyer, I. H., and Northridge, M. E., eds. 2007. *The Health of Sexual Minorities*. New York: Springer.

Moskowitz, A., Stein, J. A., and Lightfoot, M. A. 2013. The mediating role of stress and maladaptive behaviors on self-harm and suicide attempts among runaway and homeless youth. *Journal of Youth and Adolescence* 42(7): 1015–27.

Pachankis, J. E., Hatzenbuehler, M. L., Berg, R. C., Fernández-Dávila, P., Mirandola, M., Marcus, U., Weatherburn, P., and Schmidt, A. J. 2017. Anti-LGBT and anti-immigrant structural stigma: An intersectional analysis of sexual minority men's HIV risk when migrating to or within Europe. *Journal of Acquired Immune Deficiency Syndromes* 76(4): 356–66.

Raphael, D. 2003. A society in decline: The political, economic, and social determinants of health inequalities in the United States. In R. Hofrichter, ed. *Health and Social Justice: Politics, Ideology, and Inequity in the Distribution of Disease*, 59–88. San Francisco: Jossey-Bass.

Rice, E. 2013. Homelessness experiences, sexual orientation, and sexual risk taking among high school students in Los Angeles. *Journal of Adolescent Health* 52(6): 773–78.

Russell, S. T., Ryan, C., Toomey, R. B., Diaz, R. M., and Sanchez, J. 2011. Lesbian, gay, bisexual and transgender adolescent school victimization: Implications for young adult health and adjustment. *Journal of School Health* 81(5): 223–30.

Ryan, C., Huebner, D., Diaz, R. M., and Sanchez, J. 2009. Family rejection as a predictor of negative health outcomes in white and Latino lesbian, gay, and bisexual young adults. *Pediatrics* 123(1): 346–52.

Scheim, A. I., and Bauer, G. R. 2019. The Intersectional Discrimination Index: Development and validation of measures of self-reported enacted and anticipated discrimination for intercategorical analysis. *Social Science and Medicine* 226: 225–35.

Shariff-Marco, S., Gee, G. C., Breen, N., Willis, G., Reeve, B. B., Grant, D., et al. 2009. A mixed-methods approach to developing a self-reported racial/ethnic discrimination measure for use in multiethnic health surveys. *Ethnicity and Disease* 19(4): 447–53.

Strommen, E. F. 1989. "You're a what?" Family member reactions to the disclosure of homosexuality. *Journal of Homosexuality* 18(1–2): 37–58.

Sue, D. W., 2010. Microaggressions, marginality, and oppression: An introduction. In D. W. Sue, ed., *Microaggressions and Marginality*, 3–24. Hoboken, NJ: John Wiley & Sons.

Ullrich, P. M., Lutgendorf, S. K., and Stapleton, J. T. 2003. Concealment of homosexual identity, social support and CD4 cell count among HIV-seropositive gay men. *Journal of Psychosomatic Research* 54(3): 205–12.

Williams, D. R., Neighbors, H. W., and Jackson, J. S. 2003. Racial/ethnic discrimination and health: Findings from community studies. *American Journal of Public Health* 93(2): 200–208.

Williams, D. R., Yan, Y., Jackson, J. S., and Anderson, N. B. 1997. Racial differences in physical and mental health: socio-economic status, stress and discrimination. *Journal of Health Psychology* 2(3): 335–51.

Wolitski, R. J., Stall, R. D., and Valdiserri, R. O., eds. 2008. *Unequal Opportunity: Health Disparities Affecting Gay and Bisexual Men in the United States*. New York: Oxford University Press.

[ONE]

Human Rights and LGBTQ Health

Inseparable Challenges

Chris Beyrer

THE MODERN human rights movement was a response to the atrocities of World War II. The abuses of the Nazi regime, which culminated in the genocide of more than six million European Jews, the Roma, the mentally and physically disabled, homosexuals, and other persecuted minorities, shocked the conscience of the world. These fundamental violations of human life and dignity also included Nazi doctors' abuses of human subjects in a variety of medical experiments on prisoners without their consent.[1] The atrocities committed by the Japanese occupying forces in China, including medical experiments on Chinese prisoners of war, also played a role in the effort to end such violations against human beings. The medical abuses of the World War II era gave rise to the modern movement of bioethics—and the beginning of regulations that all human subjects' participation in health research must be voluntary, noncoercive, and involve participants' informed consent.[1] The immediate postwar period was marked by a great deal of activity in defining the abuses for which the world would assert "never again." These efforts culminated in the founding document of the modern human rights movement: the Universal Declaration of Human Rights (UDHR), passed by the United Nations on December 10, 1948.[2]

The US delegates to the drafting convention included former First Lady Eleanor Roosevelt and the great American historian W. E. B. Du Bois. At the time, Mrs. Roosevelt described the Universal Declaration as a "Magna Carta for all mankind."

The Declaration was, and remains, a visionary document. It was the first global attempt to define the universal rights of all persons and to define the violations of those rights. Its fundamental basis is the concept of human dignity—the dignity we all share as human beings regardless of nationality, race, religion, creed, color, age, or sex. Dignity remains the basis of human rights thinking and action. And while the concept of human dignity may vary in some cultures and contexts, the core idea—that we have a shared status as human beings and cannot be treated in ways that violate our core dignity—remains a compelling motivator for human rights advocates and for individual and communities facing the abrogation of their rights, from fighting racism and homophobia to struggling against violations of the right to speak and think freely, to vote, or to be protected from arbitrary arrest, detention without trial, torture, and extrajudicial execution.

The UDHR is a universalist document: it was intended to apply to all human beings, and not limited to the rights of citizens of a given country, or to adults, or to men as opposed to women as so many civil rights have been and continue to be limited. The UDHR, as a universalist document, included all persons living in European colonial states, which in 1948 meant virtually all Africans outside of Ethiopia and all Southeast Asians, excepting the Thais. It was also an aspirational document: it expressed a shared vision and shared goal for humanity to achieve, not a reality on the ground at the time of its framing. Professor Du Bois argued strongly, and successfully, for the prohibition of discrimination on the basis of race and ethnicity in the UDHR. Du Bois was a citizen of Louisiana, which, like virtually all of the American South in 1948, was governed by the Jim Crow statutes and by the pervasive lack of human rights protections for African Americans. Jim Crow America in 1948 was far from being free of discrimination based on race—yet the United States supported the UDHR and its aspiration for a world free of racism.

A number of the articles of the UDHR have relevance for sexual and gender minorities, and hence have implications for realizing our communities' right to health. These include:

Article 1. All persons are born free and equal in dignity and rights.

Article 2. Everyone is entitled to all the rights and freedoms without distinction of any kind, such as race, color, sex, language, religion, political or other opinion, national or social origin, property, birth or other status.

Article 7. All are equal before the law and are entitled without any discrimination to equal protection of the law.

Article 16. Men and women of full age, without any limitation due to race, nationality or religion, have the right to marry and to found a family.

Article 25. Everyone has the right to a standard of living adequate for the health and well-being of himself and of his family, including food, clothing, housing and medical care and necessary social services, and the right to security in the event of unemployment, sickness, disability, widowhood, old age or other lack of livelihood in circumstances beyond his control.

Article 25 is the first, albeit brief and general, assertion of the right to health in international human rights conventions. It defines the right to health as a component of a broader right to a minimum standard of living, which also includes the right to earn a livelihood and to have adequate housing and adequate food.

Almost no country in the world in 1948 provided full civil and human rights protections to homosexuals (as we were then generally known) or to other sexual and gender minorities. So the UDHR in practice did virtually nothing to improve the rights of LGBTQ persons in the postwar period. But like the best foundational principles, it has served as the basis for efforts to realize universal rights for all through an ever-widening expansion of what is meant by "all." This was dramatically articulated by UN Secretary-General Ban Ki-moon on Human Rights Day, December 11, 2012, which he dedicated to LGBTQ rights—a first. Secretary-General Ban's statement on that occasion quoted directly from the UDHR: "The very first article of the Universal Declaration of Human

Rights proclaims that "All human beings are born free and equal in dignity and rights." All human beings—not some, not most, but all. No one gets to decide who is entitled to human rights and who is not. . . . Let me say this loud and clear: lesbian, gay, bisexual, and transgender people are entitled to the same rights as everyone else. They, too, are born free and equal." Humanity has a long way to go to realizing this stirring vision. And for health care goals for LGBTQ persons to be achieved, such progress will be essential.

Further Advances in Human Rights

After the 1948 UDHR, little progress was made in international human rights law or treaties for several decades. This was largely due to the Cold War tensions between the Western powers and the Soviet Union and China—in particular to the tensions between the Soviet Union and the three other Western nations on the UN Security Council—the United States, Great Britain, and France. The first new conventions were both adopted in 1976. These were the International Covenant on Civil and Political Rights (ICCPR) and the International Covenant on Economic, Social and Cultural Rights (ICESCR). [3] In contrast to the Universal Declaration, these conventions were not simply aspirational but also included enforcement mechanisms, through the UN Commission on Human Rights and the office of the High Commissioner. Both of these conventions address a range of rights relevant to health and to LGBTQ populations. The right to health is generally seen as deriving from the ICESCR, and it is considered an economic and social right, not a political one.[3] Article 12 of the ICESCR lays out an explicit set of rights to health: "The States Parties to the present Covenant recognize the right of everyone to the enjoyment of the highest attainable standard of physical and mental health."[3] The "highest attainable standard" language has been used and expanded upon by countless health systems, global reports, and authors arguing for inclusion of health interventions in the "attainable standard."

Article 12 goes on to lay out four additional steps that signatory governments must undertake. The first addresses infant mortality and the well-being of the child; the second industrial hygiene; and the third and fourth are particularly important for LGBTQ health, particularly in the era of HIV/AIDS. These are "The prevention, treatment and control of epidemic, endemic and occupational and other diseases"; and "The creation of conditions which would assure to all medical service and medical attention in the event of sickness."[3] If a state is signatory to this Covenant, it has taken on a legally binding state *obligation* to respond to epidemic diseases, and to provide health care access. This has been a crucial advocacy tool for the HIV movement, and it can and should be widely used to argue for provision of health services to LGBTQ communities in any country that has signed on to the convention.

A major advance in human rights for women was the 1981 Convention on the Elimination of All Forms of Discrimination against Women (CEDAW). CEDAW includes the requirement that health services be consistent with the human rights of women and that health services ensure access to health services on basis of equality between women and men. CEDAW predates the inclusion of transgender women in the category of women, and it does not address lesbian issues. Nonetheless, like the UDHR, the Convention is a universalist document meant to be inclusive of all women and girls, and hence has the potential to be expanded.

What are the implications of a given country ratifying a covenant like CEDAW or the ICCPR? The question is fundamental to the human rights framework, and the answer includes three core elements. Each is important, each is different, and each has very different implications for actions on the part of governments, the UN, and communities in calling for human rights protections and redress for violations. The core principles are *respect, protect*, and *fulfill* the rights to which they are signatory. Signatory states must not violate these rights, and they must commit to measurable progress on their realization.

Respect for a right means essentially that a state and its agents (government officials, the police, armed forces, the courts) must not themselves be violators of the right. So a state that has ratified CEDAW cannot bar women from higher education or from the right to vote. Protecting rights is somewhat different. This means that the state is obligated to not allow any other entity within that state to violate the right. So again, if a state has signed CEDAW, it cannot allow a private-sector actor, like a company or a municipal government, to violate a protected right for women and girls. Finally, to fulfill a right, a state is committing to the gradual realization of that right. As an example, if a state has signed CEDAW, committing to equality in access to higher education for women, but data show that women account for only a small minority of graduates, the signatory state must take concrete steps to understand and address the problem until real gender equity in higher education is achieved. This can take years to decades, but the key is that measurable progress be made on fulfilling the right. Many have placed health rights in the fulfillment of rights component of the framework, recognizing that there is a gradualism inherent in trying to extend health services to all in need.

Yogyakarta, Criminalization, and Human Rights Advances

The Yogyakarta Principles of 2006 were a major advance in the human rights specific to LGBTQ communities. Named for the Indonesian city where the principles were drafted, the Yogyakara Principles were a visionary attempt to review all of the existing human rights laws and conventions and their application in relation to sexual orientation and gender identity.[4] In all, the Principles identified 29 domains of international human rights law and convention with relevance to LGBTQ rights. A shortlist of these rights included that LGBTQ persons have the right to the universal enjoyment of human rights (principle 1); the right to equality and nondiscrimination (principle 2); the right to recognition before the law (principle 3); the right to life (principle 4); the right to security of the person (principle 5); the right to privacy; and the right to freedom from torture, cruel, inhuman, or degrading treatment (principle 10).[4]

The realization of the rights in the Yogyakarta Principles is the goal of many in the international human rights community and of LGBTQ communities facing persecution worldwide. The principles lay out a clear case for extending full rights and protections to LGBTQ persons.

However, the reality for many is radically different—and indeed, deteriorating in many countries. LGBTQ individuals, couples, families, and communities remain criminalized in some 75 countries worldwide. More than half of the African countries, some of which report the highest HIV prevalence rates in the world, continue to criminalize same-sex behavior between consenting adults. In the most extreme case of rights abrogation—the right to life itself—11 states impose the death penalty for same-sex relations between consenting adults in some or all of their territories. These include Yemen, Pakistan, Saudi Arabia, Iran, the states in Nigeria governed by sharia law, and Sudan.[5] The emergence of the Islamic State in Syria and Iraq has added a new nonstate actor to the list of regimes executing people for known or suspected homosexuality.[6] Jessica Stern, the executive director of OutRight Action International, told the UN Security Council that courts established by ISIS in Iraq and Syria claimed to have punished sodomy with stoning, firing squads, and beheadings and by pushing men from tall buildings.[6]

OutRight Action International has also documented the export of extremist anti-LGBTQ ideology by US evangelical Christian conservatives to many African states and to the Russian Federation.[7] US evangelical leaders, including Scott Lively and Don Schmierer, have conducted seminars in Uganda, a particular target country for these activities, and have been involved in the drafting of Uganda's harsh anti-gay law.[8] In an important advance for human rights in Uganda, Lively was indicted for crimes against humanity for his promotion of anti-LGBTQ activities in two US courts (in Maryland and Massachusetts). He has since run for governor of Massachusetts. Both cases were brought forward by courageous LGBTQ activists in Uganda, led by Sexual Minorities Uganda, and have argued that Lively was violating the human rights of LGBTQ Ugandans.[8]

A major victory in human rights for LGBTQ persons was the 1994 UN Human Rights Committee decision in a case known as *Toonen v. Australia*. *Toonen* was the first recognition of gay and lesbian rights within the UN human rights system. The case originated in the Australian province of Tasmania, which alone among Australia's states territories continued to criminalize same-sex behavior. Failing to overturn the law, the plaintiff's attorneys took the case to the UN Human Rights Committee, arguing that the plaintiff's basic human rights were being violated by the Tasmanian law. The case was argued on the principles of privacy rights and equality rights. Article 17 of the International Covenant on Civil and Political Rights, to which Australia was signatory, bars "arbitrary or unlawful interference" with privacy. Article 26 of the same statute prohibits discrimination "on any ground such as race, color, sex, language, religion, political or other opinion, national or social origin, property, birth or other status." In *Toonen*, the UN ruled that "sex" in the statute included sexual orientation, and hence Tasmania could not discriminate against its citizens on the basis of sexual orientation.[9]

Since *Toonen*, a number of courts have used the ruling to bolster the case for LGBTQ rights. These include India's repeal of its sodomy laws in 2009 (now reversed) and the repeal of these laws in Nepal in 2010. Other treaty bodies within the United Nations now also deal with sexual orientation issues. The UN Human Rights Committee has repeatedly concluded that laws criminalizing same-sex sodomy constitute discrimination based on sexual orientation. The UN Committee on Torture and the UN Working Group on Arbitrary Detention condemned Egypt's gender-neutral "debauchery" law as constituting discrimination on the basis of sexual orientation. And the UN Committee on the Rights of the Child has analyzed disparities in age-of-consent laws between same- and different-sex partners as sexual orientation discrimination.

The United States during the Obama Administration reversed a decades-long US policy and included LGBTQ rights in its policies and diplomacy. Secretary of State Hillary Rodham Clinton articulated the new US policy in a major speech at the UN Commission on Human Rights in Geneva in December 2011: "Gay rights are human rights, and human rights are gay rights."[10] The United States now provides the opportunity to seek political asylum on the basis of persecution for sexual orientation and gender identity, and it has welcomed LGBTQ rights activists from a number of African and Caribbean nations where they were in danger.

The Global Commission on HIV and the Law in 2012 reviewed laws criminalizing consensual adult same-sex relations and found that they undermined effective HIV programming for gay, bisexual, and other men who have sex with men (MSM).[11] This report was an important step in that it explicitly linked LGBTQ human rights to health outcomes.

LGBTQ Rights and Health Activism

The movement for LGBTQ human rights and for LGBTQ health can be said to have been driven by the terrible urgencies of the emerging HIV pandemic in the early 1980s. HIV changed the lives of gay men and our allies forever, and it has had profound and lasting impacts on LGBTQ human rights and on health.[12] From the epidemic's beginning, gay men, lesbians, and their nongay allies were at the forefront of AIDS advocacy and service delivery, fighting for resources, legal changes, and research. Gay men were involved in advancing the research agenda on every front from epidemiology to prevention, from treatment to public policy.[12] The extent to which early LGBTQ rights and the gay men's and MSM movements arose from local contexts and histories is striking. As an example, the Brazilian gay activist group Grupo Pela Vidda grew out of the civil-society movement for restoration of democracy and human rights and against military rule in Brazil. The group then led the early civil-society response demanding treatment access for HIV in the country—which subsequently became the first low- or middle-income country to commit to universal antiviral drug access; Brazil remains a leader in HIV responses today.[12] In contrast, in South Africa, Tseko Simon Nkoli typified the social movement that fought to end apartheid in South Africa and to increase the rights and recognition of LGBTQ communities.[12] South Africa became the first (and still only) African country to include LGBTQ rights in its constitution and to have marriage equality for same-sex couples; it remains among the few countries willing to provide comprehensive HIV care for gay and other MSM in publicly funded clinics.[12]

In the United States, Brazil, and South Africa the HIV movements were spurred and radicalized by the inaction of governments.[12] Frustration with inaction by governments led gay men and others to forge a new style of AIDS activism that was political, confrontational, and visible—best exemplified by ACT UP (the AIDS Coalition to Unleash Power), which recognized the connection between government neglect and homophobia during the Reagan Administration.[12] ACT UP and an array of other advocacy and activist groups helped transform the HIV response, and they continue to inform other movements for health equity. The results of this activism included speeding regulatory approval of products for expanded clinical research, lowering the price of licensed HIV medicines, and creating legislation to fund HIV programs and services.[13]

In much of the world, however, the human cost of advocacy has been terribly high. LGBTQ and HIV rights activists have faced significant backlash, and activists and advocates alike have been beaten, arrested, and killed. Among gay men murdered for their pioneering leadership are Alim Mongoche in Cameroon, Steve Harvey in Jamaica, David Kato in Uganda, and Thapelo Makutle in South Africa. For every arrest and murder that is public, there are surely hundreds that will never be known or reported. Arrests and murders highlight that the struggle is far from won and that comprehensive HIV prevention and treatment cannot yet be achieved in these contexts. Lesbian women and transgender individuals have likewise faced brutality, intimidation, threats, and extrajudicial killings. In several African states, lesbian women and transgender men have been brutalized by the crime known as "corrective rape."[14] While many of these horrific abuses, including the murder of activists and corrective rape, are clearly crimes, they become human rights issues if states fail to investigate and prosecute these crimes. Impunity for crimes is a failure to protect human rights and a failure to fulfill those rights. No one has been charged with the murders of the four men named above, and the states involved are culpable at a minimum for a failure to protect.

LGBTQ Human Rights and Health Research

What is the future of health research and LGBTQ human rights? One conceptual pathway that many groups are exploring is to frame human rights as understudied social determinants of health. An example of this kind of work is research done by my own group and others on the impact of human rights violations on measurable health outcomes. In the HIV model, which has high relevance due to the very marked health disparity in HIV burden and risks experienced by gay, bisexual and other MSM and among transgender women who have sex with men, this work has included qualitative, quantitative, epidemiologic, clinical, and health policy research on the impact of rights violations, including discrimination on health care access for the populations in HIV programs.[15-17]

Many investigators see human rights as structural determinants of health, overlapping considerably with the framing of stigma and discrimination.[18-20] This work is increasingly adding biomarkers, such as HIV viral load, or incident HIV infection, to assess the tangible impacts of rights violations, or protections, on clinical outcomes. An outstanding example is work by Sheree Schwartz and colleagues working with MSM in Nigeria before and after that country's adoption of an extreme antihomosexuality law, which demonstrated a measurable increase in viral load among the HIV community after the law's adoption.[18]

The next phases of health research and human rights work for LGBTQ populations will likely focus on assessing the impact of interventions in the human rights area, including rights protections, on health outcomes. The demonstration of measurable benefits to health in protecting and improving rights outcomes for LGBTQ communities is an exciting task awaiting the coming generation of health and rights researchers. The research agenda around the health impacts of marriage equality for same-sex couples in one example of this kind of work. The health benefits of the state recognition of transgender identities is another. This is an important but until now markedly understudied area. But the connections between human rights and health outcomes are increasingly becoming clear. It is now imperative to use the rights framework to improve the health, well-being, and human rights realities for LGBTQ persons and communities worldwide.

References

1. Lifton, R. J. 1986. *The Nazi Doctors: Medical Killing and the Psychology of Genocide.* New York: HarperCollins.

2. Universal Declaration of Human Rights, https://www.un.org/en/universal-declaration-human-rights/

3. Marks, S. P., ed. 2012. *Health and Human Rights: Basic International Documents* (Cambridge, MA: Harvard University Press), 5–13

4. The Yogyakarta Principles are published at www.yogyakartaprinciples.org /principles_en.htm.

5. The International Lesbian and Gay Association (ILGA: ilga.org), regularly tracks the status of LGBT laws globally. See Lucas Ramon Mendos, *State-Sponsored Homophobia 2019: Global Legislation Overview Update* (Geneva: ILGA, December 2019). OutRight Action International (https://outrightinternational.org/), formerly the International Lesbian and Gay Human Rights Commission, also actively documents the status of rights for LGBT communities.

6. Associated Press. "Islamic State has killed at least 30 people for sodomy, UN told." August 25, 2015.

7. ILGHRC Statement: "Uganda: The U.S. religious right exports homophobia to Africa." March 4, 2009.

8. Beyrer, C. 2014. Pushback: The current wave of anti-homosexuality laws and impacts on health. *PLoS Med* 11(6): e1001658.

9. *Toonen v. Australia*, Communication No. 488/1992, UN Doc CCPR/C/50/D/ 488/1992 (1994).

10. Remarks of US Secretary of State Hillary Rodham Clinton in recognition of International Human Rights Day at the Palais des Nations, Geneva, Switzerland, December 6, 2011.

11. United Nations Development Program. Global Commission on HIV and the Law (New York: UNDP, 2012), www.hivlawcommission.org.

12. Trapence, G., Collins, C., Avrett, S., Carr, R., Sanchez, H., Ayala, G., Diouf, D., Beyrer, C., and Baral, S. D. 2012. From personal survival to public health: Community leadership by men who have sex with men in the response to HIV. *Lancet* 380 (9839): 400–410.

13. Beyrer, C., Sullivan, P. S., Sanchez, J., Dowdy, D., Altman, D., Trapence, G., Collins, C., Katabira, E., Kazatchkine, M., Sidibe, M., and Mayer, K. H. 2012. A call to action for comprehensive HIV services for men who have sex with men. *Lancet* 380 (9839): 424–38.

14. Carter, C. The brutality of "corrective rape." *New York Times*, July 27, 2013.

15. Baral, S., Trapence, G., Motimedi, F., Umar, E., Iipinge, S., Dausab, F., and Beyrer, C. 2009. HIV prevalence risks for HIV infection, and human rights among men who have sex with men (MSM) in Malawi, Namibia, and Botswana. *PLoS One* 4(3): e4997.

16. Fay, H., Baral, S. D., Trapence, G., Motimedi, F., Umar, E., Iipinge, S., Dausab, F., Wirtz, A., and Beyrer, C. 2010. Stigma, health care access, and HIV knowledge among men who have sex with men in Malawi, Namibia, and Botswana. *AIDS and Behavior* 15(6): 1088–97.

17. Baral, S., Adams, D., Lebona, J., Kaibe, B., Letsie, P., Tshehlo, R., Wirtz, A., and Beyrer, C. 2011. A cross-sectional assessment of population demographics, HIV risks and human rights contexts among men who have sex with men in Lesotho. *Journal of the International AIDS Society* 14(1): 36.

18. Poteat, T., Diouf, D., Drame, F. M., Ndaw, M., Traore, C., Dhaliwal, M., Beyrer, C., and Baral, S. 2011. HIV risk among MSM in Senegal: A qualitative rapid assessment of the impact of enforcing laws that criminalize same sex practices. *PLoS One* 6(12): e28760.

19. Semugoma, P., Beyrer, C., and Baral, S. 2012. Assessing the effects of anti-homosexuality legislation in Uganda on HIV prevention, treatment, and care services. *SAHARA J: Journal of the Social Aspects of HIV/AIDS* 9 (3): 173–77.

20. Wirtz, A. L., Zelaya, C. E., Peryshkina, A., Latkin, C., Mogilnyi, V., Galai, N., Dyakonov K., and Beyrer C. 2014. Social and structural risks for HIV among migrant and immigrant men who have sex with men in Moscow, Russia: Implications for prevention. *AIDS Care* 26(3): 387–95.

21. Schwartz, S. R., Nowak, R. G., Orazulike, I., Keshinro, B., Ake, J., Kennedy, S., Njoku, O., Blattner, W. A., Charurat, M. E., Baral, S. D., and TRUST Study Group. 2015. The immediate effect of the Same-Sex Marriage Prohibition Act on stigma, discrimination, and engagement on HIV prevention and treatment services in men who have sex with men in Nigeria: Analysis of prospective data from the TRUST cohort. *Lancet HIV* 2(7): e299–e306

TWO

Global Health/LGBTQ Health

Tonia Poteat and Shauna Stahlman

SEXUAL DIVERSITY is ubiquitous throughout the animal kingdom and across human cultures. Anthropological and literary evidence suggest that this same-sex sexuality and variations in gender identity and expression have existed as far back as there are human records. Although the World Health Organization declassified homosexuality as an illness or disorder in 1990, and despite a widespread consensus among scientists that homosexuality is a natural and normal variation of human sexuality, same-sex relationships remain illegal in roughly 75 countries. These discriminatory laws facilitate stigma toward LGBTQ individuals and impede progress in attaining public health goals by increasing the burden of mental health and causing fear and avoidance of health care seeking.

Despite continued challenges, the twenty-first century has been remarkable for the ways in which sexual and gender minorities are organizing communities, identities, family structures, and social movements on a global basis. Globalization, fostered by advances in communication technologies and social media, has led to rapid changes in the visibility of LGBTQ populations around the world. Sexual and gender minorities can now access online communities that may foster a stronger sense of sexual and gender identity. In this context, local categories for sexuality and gender sit alongside or are even subsumed by identities previously seen as exclusively Western. For example, Thai male same-sex behavior was historically constituted in a masculine-feminine dichotomy, with little to no recognition of masculine men together as a couple. Modern Thai culture now includes communities of out gay men and transgender communities who see themselves as quite separate. These new identities challenge previously held social norms, old constructs of gender, and even national identities.

In stigmatizing social environments, LGBTQ community groups have taken leading roles in providing HIV and sexual health services to gay men and other men who have sex with men (MSM). These programs also provide social support to LGBTQ and broader communities in the form of social capital by strengthening bonds between group members; increasing availability of emotional, financial, and other resources through social networks; and improving perceptions of trustworthiness of others and the ability to work together to solve problems facing the community. Newly formed LGBTQ organizations may provide not only social and emotional support, but also foundations for community health services and human rights advocacy. Examples include the Coalition for African Lesbians, Global Action for Trans Equality, the Global Forum for MSM and HIV, the Council for Global Equality, and others. These organizations and others undertake their efforts during a tumultuous period for LGBTQ rights.

Substantial biological evidence supports the diversity of human sexuality, including genetic, neurohormonal, and socio-behavioral research. However, research regarding human sexuality needs to be much more widely disseminated and discussed in the public domain, and incorporated by governments and policymakers when building new legislation. On the one hand, same-sex couples are able to legally marry in South Africa and the United States; recognition of a third gender is legal in Nepal; and a group of transgender women in Argentina have won their legal case for reparations for lifetime experiences of stigma and discrimination. On the other hand, employment discrimination on the basis of gender identity or sexual orientation is still legal in the United States.

Russia, Ukraine, Nigeria, and other countries continue to press for and enact antihomosexuality legislation. Discriminatory policies facilitate stigma and violence against sexual and gender minorities, contributing to the global burden of sexual identity stigma that is already common in most parts of the world. This complex, rapidly changing world is the context in which we approach attempts to understand and improve LGBTQ health globally.

Global health has traditionally focused on maternal child health, child survival, and infectious diseases with little attention to LGBTQ issues. The HIV crisis opened one path to addressing LGBTQ health globally, particularly among gay, bisexual, and men who have sex with men; these changing social and sexual networks have influenced the epidemiology of HIV and sexually transmitted infectious diseases (STIs). However, the time has come to address LGBTQ health issues distinct from HIV. Research among LGBTQ communities in high-income countries suggests that sexual and gender minorities experience significant health disparities beyond HIV, including increased risk for suicide and homelessness among LGBTQ youth; higher risk of STIs among gay men and other MSM; increased likelihood of being overweight or obese among lesbians and bisexual women; reduced uptake of preventive health care services among lesbians and bisexual women; increased isolation and lack of social services among elderly LGBTQ individuals; higher risk of victimization, mental health issues, and suicide among transgender individuals; and higher rates of tobacco, alcohol, and other drug use among the general LGBTQ population.[1] It is likely that LGBTQ populations in low- and middle-income countries experience similar health disparities as well as disparities associated with poverty and poor health infrastructure. Determining the health status of sexual and gender minorities internationally and addressing pressing health disparities is a critical task for global health workers.

What Do We Know?

Understanding the global state of research among gender and sexual minorities is a daunting task, complicated by diverse and evolving global identities, geographic variation, and language limitations. However, recent published literature provides a snapshot of areas where research has taken place and helps to identify gaps in our knowledge. Health research among sexual minorities has focused on three main topics: sexual health, psychosocial health, and more recently, structural violence.

Sexual Health: HIV and STIs

The global health literature as it relates to sexual and gender minorities is highly focused on HIV among gay, bisexual, and other men who have sex with men. Of 843 citations retrieved in a literature search of health among gender and sexual minorities outside Europe and the United States spanning the period 2011–2015, more than 600 (greater than 80%) were about HIV. Most of this research operationalizes sexual identity as MSM, subsuming gay and bisexual-identified men within this category, and often excluding transgender men who have sex with men and/or conflating transgender women who have sex with men. Most data that do exist on sexual minorities and HIV are concentrated in high-income countries; however, there is a growing literature on HIV among MSM in low- and middle-income countries.

In almost every country, MSM experience disproportionate vulnerability to HIV compared with other men and with the general population.[2] These disparities have been linked to a multidimensional array of factors, including risks at the individual, network, community, and structural levels.[3] For example, biological and behavioral risks such as condomless anal sex increase risk at the individual level. Sex role versatility further enhances the spread of HIV at the network level by enabling MSM who are newly infected through receptive anal sex to then transmit HIV efficiently to new partners when they are insertive. Sexual behavior or identity stigma toward MSM at the community level can limit the provision and uptake of HIV prevention, treatment, and care services and reduce health-seeking behaviors. Finally, at the structural level, discriminatory policies such as the criminalization of same-sex practices in many countries present significant barriers to HIV prevention and have been associated with higher levels of violence and stigma against MSM.

Emerging data on HIV among transgender women reveal even greater health disparities.[4] Primary drivers of the burden of HIV among transgender women, similar to MSM, relate to biological, network-level, community-level, and structural-level factors.[5] Stigma, social exclusion, and economic marginalization lead to high prevalence of sex work among transgender women.[6] These factors, coupled with the increased transmission probability of condomless anal sex, likely contribute to increased risk. However, HIV prevalence data among transgender women are virtually absent from Africa and Eastern Europe–Central Asia. In addition, there is a general lack of research regarding the HIV risk behaviors and sexual health needs of transgender men. The limited data on sexual health among lesbians, bisexual women, and other women who have sex with women (WSW) also point to possible HIV disparities[7] as well as associations between sexual health disparities and multilevel stigma.[8]

CASE STUDY: SEXUAL HEALTH AMONG LESBIAN, BISEXUAL, QUEER, AND WOMEN WHO HAVE SEX WITH WOMEN

A recent review of the literature on sexual health of WSW in low- and middle-income countries found wide variety in the types of information reported as well as in the prevalence of STIs and HIV.[7] Despite a widely held belief that WSW are at low risk of acquiring and transmitting STIs and HIV, it was determined that many WSW engage in sexual behaviors, including exchange of bodily fluids, that could transmit STIs or HIV to female partners. The review also indicated that there are no standards for safer sex among WSW, and WSW report infrequent use of protective barriers such as condoms or dental dams with both male and female partners. Greater effort should be put forth to include WSW in the global HIV response effort.

Psychosocial: Mental Health, Substance Use

Mental health disparities, particularly related to depression and suicide, have been found consistently among sexual and gender minority populations around the world.[9-12] Most of this research has explored suicidal ideation and attempts by adolescent sexual minorities, with little international data on other groups. While sexual and gender minorities are more likely to experience poor mental health, we also see evidence that social support and psychological counseling can be effective in reducing psychological distress.[11]

According to a 2011 Institute of Medicine report on the health of LGBT people, LGB adults have higher rates of smoking, alcohol use, and substance use than heterosexual adults. One potential explanation points to the minority stress model, in which LGBTQ people use substances in order to cope with increased levels of stigma including family rejection. Cigarette smoking is more prevalent among LGB populations than among heterosexual populations across the globe.[13] However, the disparities in alcohol use seen in the United States may not exist in other parts of the world.[14,15] Use of hormones, soft-tissue fillers, and other gender-affirming substances without medical supervision is common among transgender populations globally.[16–18] Data gaps exist for smoking, alcohol, and drug use among transgender populations outside of North America.

CASE STUDY: DRUG USE AMONG GAY MEN AND OTHER MSM IN ASIA

An online survey of 10,861 MSM recruited from 12 different countries throughout Asia compared patterns of illicit drug use by participants' HIV status.[19] MSM living with HIV reported overall higher levels of individual drug use and polydrug use than those who were not aware they were living with HIV. In this sample, stimulant drug use was associated with identifying as gay, having more gay friends, having more casual male sex partners, and living with HIV. Overall findings suggest a consistent and similar pattern of drug use among some networks of gay men in Asia, as has been observed in other regions of the world. These patterns of drug use and abuse pose a clear risk to the health of gay men and other MSM, including risk for HIV seroconversion.

Structural and Physical Violence: Stigma, Discrimination, Victimization, and Minority Stress

LGBTQ populations experience gender- and sexuality-related stigma and discrimination that lead to minority stress, compounded by intersecting stigmatized identities along lines of race, ethnicity, age, gender, gender presentation, social class, ability, and more. The effects of minority stress are related to the health disparities we see in stigmatized populations. Stigma may be linked to HIV infection indirectly through depression, substance use, and access to HIV prevention services. More directly, stigma leads to violence and victimization, especially against transgender and gender nonconforming individuals.

An emerging body of literature has addressed the impact of minority stress on sexual and gender minorities internationally. Studies in the Middle East and North Africa[20,21] and sub-Saharan Africa[22] have found that minority stress is associated with poorer mental and physical health among LGB populations, with some evidence that poor mental health mediates the relationship between minority stress and physical health.[20] High levels of sexual behavior stigma may also lead to LGBTQ sexual and romantic partnerships being conducted in secrecy, which can promote sexual risk behaviors and unsupportive relationships.[23] Cross-cultural studies have found that strong social networks may help to ameliorate the negative effects of both internalized homophobia and external homophobic discrimination.[24]

Physical, psychological, sexual, and structural violence against gender and sexual minorities has been documented in every region of the world.[25–28] Sexual assault perpetrated with the intent to change the victim's sexual orientation or gender identity and punish same-sex attraction has received the most attention among lesbians in South Africa.[29] However, evidence is emerging that so-called corrective rape takes place in other countries[30] and against men as well.[31,32] In addition to the harm caused by violence itself, experiences of violence affect the psychological and physical well-being of survivors.

Harassment and violence against transgender people are well documented and ubiquitous.[33,34] In addition, growing attention is being paid to the health impacts (increased risk of HIV and suicide) of structural violence such as barriers to gender-affirming health care and lack of appropriate gender-congruent identity documents.[35] Evidence suggests that intervening to address transphobia at structural and interpersonal levels can reduce transgender health disparities.[36]

Case Study: High Prevalence of Violence against Transgender Women in Brazil

Data were analyzed from a respondent-driven sampling study of 304 transgender women in Brazil.[37] This study found that more than half of participants reported being a victim of violence (65%), and a majority also reported being a victim of homophobia and/or transphobia (89%). Receiving money in exchange for sex was also common, with 66% exchanging sex for money in the last 30 days and 87% in a lifetime. These results illustrate the disproportionate burden of stigma, discrimination, and violence against transgender women. In addition, social and economic marginalization contribute to transgender women engaging in survival sex work, thereby putting them at risk for HIV and other adverse health outcomes.

What Do We Need to Know?

Gaps clearly remain in the scientific literature on global LGBTQ Health. The vast majority of international studies have taken place among men. In particular, international data on health among bisexual people and/or transgender people are sparse. Few international studies have teased apart the dimensions of sexual orientation (attraction, behavior, identity); nor have they addressed intersectionality within LGBTQ populations and the implications for how best to address health disparities. We need a global research agenda that addresses the spectrum of LGBTQ ages and identities and fills the gaps in our knowledge beyond HIV. Importantly, we need to build our knowledge of resilience and coping strategies that can inform effective interventions to prevent illness and improve health for gender and sexual minorities around the globe.

Why Do We Need This Information?

While a preponderance of data derive from high-income countries, the vast majority of the world's population lives in low- and middle-income countries. Currently available research points to health disparities that may be only the tip of the iceberg. In a global world interconnected by the internet, travel, and interdependent economies, we must explore and address health disparities worldwide. We cannot address LGBTQ health in the absence of a global health research agenda that includes facing the threats that homophobia and transphobia present. Global health is a core competency for LGBTQ health.

What Can Public Health Researchers Do?

Reducing global LGBTQ health disparities can seem a formidable task. However, it can be done. While health disparities might seem a depressing area of research, funding often follows a clear and irrefutable demonstration of evidence or, as is commonly said, "dollars follow data." Health policymakers rely on researchers to produce actionable data. Researchers may also partner with international LGBTQ organizations to provide data they need to support their advocacy work. Community-based participatory action research is one key approach to partnerships between researchers and activists. This type of research lends itself to multidisciplinary approaches that are common in public health and are designed to lead to change.

Inevitably, there will be barriers to international LGBTQ research, including limited research capacity of local organizations, limited funding, and lack of political will. However, these barriers can be overcome. Organizations like amfAR and the US Department of State's Global Equality Fund have supported small community-based LGBTQ organizations to build their capacity for advocacy and research. These local organizations, in partnership with funders, are best positioned to address the specific political context in their country or region. Engaging global and local LGBTQ communities and adapting research approaches to the specific context are critical to success.

Training health professionals to improve competency when caring for LGBTQ populations is essential. Providers should be able to provide adequate health information to LGBTQ clients in addition to providing comprehensive, safe, and appropriate services. Specific guidance on promoting the health of LGBTQ individuals in their communities may be necessary for providers to fulfill their ethical obligation to serve all people seeking care.

More data are needed for a better understanding of the health needs of all LGBTQ persons, particularly among low- and middle-income countries. Collecting and analyzing a repository of data on LGBTQ health across the globe, even if it does not include primary data, would provide an extremely useful resource for local LGBTQ organizations. Finally, developing training resources for new generations of LGBTQ researchers to address the health needs of gender and sexual minorities, globally, is urgently needed.

References

1. World Health Organization. 2013. *Improving the Health and Well-being of Lesbian, Gay, Bisexual and Transgender Persons.*

2. Beyrer C., Sullivan, P., Sanchez, J., et al. 2013. The increase in global HIV epidemics in MSM. *AIDS* 27(17): 2665–78.

3. Baral S., Logie, C. H., Grosso, A., Wirtz, A. L., and Beyrer, C. 2013. Modified social ecological model: A tool to guide the assessment of the risks and risk contexts of HIV epidemics. *BMC Public Health* 13: 482.

4. Baral S. D., Poteat, T., Strömdahl, S., Wirtz, A. L., Guadamuz, T. E., and Beyrer, C. 2013. Worldwide burden of HIV in transgender women: A systematic review and meta-analysis. *The Lancet Infectious Diseases* 13(3): 214–22.

5. Poteat, T., Reisner, S. L., and Radix, A. 2014. HIV epidemics among transgender women. *Current Opinion in HIV and AIDS* 9 (2): 168–73.

6. Poteat, T., Wirtz, A. L., Radix, A., et al. 2015. HIV risk and preventive interventions in transgender women sex workers. *Lancet* 385 (9964): 274–86.

7. Tat, S. A., Marrazzo, J. M., and Graham, S. M. 2015. Women who have sex with women living in low- and middle-income countries: A systematic review of sexual health and risk behaviors. *LGBT Health* 2 (2): 91–104.

8. Poteat T. C., Logie, C. H., Adams, D., et al. 2015. Stigma, sexual health, and human rights among women who have sex with women in Lesotho. *Reproductive Health Matters* 23(46): 107–16.

9. Yadegarfard, M., Ho, R., and Bahramabadian, F. 2013. Influences on loneliness, depression, sexual-risk behaviour and suicidal ideation among Thai transgender youth. *Culture, Health, and Sexuality* 15(6): 726–37.

10. Ghorayeb, D.B., and Dalgalarrondo, P. Homosexuality: Mental health and quality of life in a Brazilian socio-cultural context. *International Journal of Social Psychology* 57(5): 496–500.

11. Yang, F, Li, L., Yang, S. X., et al. 2012. [Mental health situation of men who have sex with men among university students]. *Zhonghua Liu Xing Bing Xue Za Zhi* 33(11): 1139–40.

12. Horton, P. 2014. "I thought I was the only one": The misrecognition of LGBT youth in contemporary Vietnam. *Culture, Health, and Sexuality* 16(8): 960–73.

13. Berg, C. J., Nehl, E. J., Wong, F. Y., et al. 2011. Prevalence and correlates of tobacco use among a sample of MSM in Shanghai, China. *Nicotine and Tobaccco Research* 13(1): 22–28.

14. Bloomfield, K., Wicki, M., Wilsnack, S., Hughes, T., and Gmel, G. 2011. International differences in alcohol use according to sexual orientation. *Journal of Substance Abuse* 32(4): 210–19.

15. Yu, F., Nehl, E. J., Zheng, T., et al. 2013. A syndemic including cigarette smoking and sexual risk behaviors among a sample of MSM in Shanghai, China. *Drug and Alcohol Dependence* 132(1–2): 265–70.

16. Gooren, L. J., Sungkaew, T., and Giltay, E. J. 2013. Exploration of functional health, mental well-being and cross-sex hormone use in a sample of Thai male-to-female transgendered persons (kathoeys). *Asian Journal of Andrology* 15(2): 280–85.

17. Hardon A., Idrus, N. I., and Hymans, T. D. 2013. Chemical sexualities: The use of pharmaceutical and cosmetic products by youth in South Sulawesi, Indonesia. *Reproductive Health Matters* 21(41): 214–24.

18. Poompruek, P., Boonmongkon, P., and Guadamuz, T. E. 2014. "For me . . . it's a miracle": Injecting beauty among *kathoeis* in a provincial Thai city. *International Journal of Drug Policy* 25(4): 798–803.

19. Wei, C., Guadamuz, T. E., Lim, S.H., Huang, Y., and Koe, S. 2012. Patterns and levels of illicit drug use among men who have sex with men in Asia. *Drug and Alcohol Dependence* 120(1): 246–49.

20. Shilo, G., and Mor, Z. 2014. The impact of minority stressors on the mental and physical health of lesbian, gay, and bisexual youths and young adults. *Health and Social Work*. 39(3): 161–71.

21. Wagner, G. J., Aunon, F. M., Kaplan, R. L., et al. 2013. Sexual stigma, psychological well-being and social engagement among men who have sex with men in Beirut, Lebanon. *Culture, Health, and Sexuality* 15(5): 570–82.

22. McAdams-Mahmoud, A., R. Stephenson, C. Rentsch, et al. 2014. Minority stress in the lives of men who have sex with men in Cape Town, South Africa. *Journal of Homosexuality* 61(6): 847–67.

23. Stahlman, S., Bechtold, K., Sweitzer, S., et al. 2015. Sexual identity stigma and social support among men who have sex with men in Lesotho: A qualitative analysis. *Reproductive Health Matters* 23(46): 127–35.

24. Chard, A. N., Finneran, C., Sullivan, P. S., and Stephenson, R. 2015. Experiences of homophobia among gay and bisexual men: Results from a cross-sectional study in seven countries. *Culture, Health, and Sexuality* 17(10): 1–16.

25. Elouard, Y., and Essen, B. 2013. Psychological violence experienced by men who have sex with men in Puducherry, India: A qualitative study. *Journal of Homosexuality* 60 (11): 1581–1601.

26. Wong, Y. 2012. Islam, sexuality, and the marginal positioning of Pengkids and their girlfriends in Malaysia. *Journal of Lesbian Studies* 16(4): 435–48.

27. Smith, R. 2015. Healthcare experiences of lesbian and bisexual women in Cape Town, South Africa. *Culture, Health, and Sexuality* 17(2):180–93.

28. Mavhandu-Mudzusi, A. H., and Sandy, P. T. 2015. Religion-related stigma and discrimination experienced by lesbian, gay, bisexual and transgender students at a South African rural-based university. *Culture, Health, and Sexuality* 17(8):1049–56.

29. Brown, R. 2012. Corrective rape in South Africa: A continuing plight despite an international human rights response. *Annual Survey of International and Comparative Law* 18: 45–66.

30. Victims of corrective rape speak up. *The Times of India*, June 10, 2015.

31. Latypov A., Rhodes, T., and Reynolds, L. 2013. Prohibition, stigma and violence against men who have sex with men: effects on HIV in Central Asia. *Central Asian Survey* 32(1): 52–65.

32. Sabidó, M., Kerr, L. R. F. S., Mota, R. S., et al. 2015. Sexual violence against men who have sex with men in Brazil: A respondent-driven sampling survey. *AIDS and Behavior* 2015:1–12.

33. Stotzer, R. L. Violence against transgender people: A review of United States data. 2009. *Aggression and Violent Behavior* 14(3):170–79.

34. Byrne, J. 2013. *Transgender Health and Human Rights*. United Nations Development Programme.

35. Poteat, T., Wirtz, A. L., Radix, A., et al. 2014. HIV risk and preventive interventions in transgender women sex workers. *Lancet* 385 (6736): 274–86.

36. Bauer, G. R., Scheim, A. I., Pyne, J., Travers, R., and Hammond, R. 2015. Intervenable factors associated with suicide risk in transgender persons: A respondent-driven sampling study in Ontario, Canada. *BMC Public Health* 15: 525.

37. Martins, T. A., Kerr, L. R., Macena, R. H., et al. 2013. *Travestis*, an unexplored population at risk of HIV in a large metropolis of northeast Brazil: A respondent-driven sampling survey. *AIDS Care* 25(5): 606–12.

THREE

A Love Note to Future Generations of LGBTQ Health Researchers

Ron Stall, Chris Beyrer, Tonia Poteat, Brian Dodge, and José A. Bauermeister

THE HISTORICAL record yields abundant evidence to show that research on LGBTQ populations has deep historical roots within industrialized countries. Notably, the historical record shows that important research efforts were begun even during periods in which support for research on the health of LGBTQ populations was minimal or even actively suppressed. This general theme is also found in the description of LGBTQ research conducted in low- and middle-income country settings, where activists and researchers have documented many dangerous health disparities within sexual minority populations, perhaps linked to the very adverse social conditions in which they reside. It is also clear that with globalization distinct LGBTQ communities are emerging in diverse cultures all over the world. From the evidence that is available to us so far, it is also likely that these communities are suffering from dangerous health disparities in contexts that offer them few resources to address these problems. Chapter 2 offers a set of conceptual tools to work for structural changes so that LGBTQ communities across the globe can have access to the tools that they require to combat and resolve the many health disparities that we know already exist among these populations.

Thus, the current state of research in LGBTQ health is full of promise based on recent progress not only in terms of civil rights for LGBTQ populations in the industrialized countries, but also in terms of the substantial progress that has been made to describe and even to start to address the many different health disparities suffered by LGBTQ populations in the industrialized West. However, this is also a period of daunting challenges: the health research that has been done has overwhelmingly focused on men who have sex with men in the industrialized countries and has underinvested in research on the health needs of lesbian women, bisexual men and women, transgender populations, and intersex people. Furthermore, while funding has focused on the control of sexually transmitted infectious diseases, research to develop interventions that address noninfectious diseases, psychosocial health problems, and social pathologies such as violence victimization has been underemphasized. Even more challenging is the fact that as sexual minority communities become more established in countries around the globe, the many different known LGBTQ health disparities documented in the existing literature and those that may be specific to particular cultural contexts could become intractable health challenges over time.

This expansive agenda cannot be completed in a few years: rather it will take many decades, if not generations, of concerted effort to realize. That said, this research agenda is as ambitious as it is exciting, and it offers investigators many opportunities to make groundbreaking contributions in the provision of health care to marginalized communities. The work will need to begin by mapping the extent of the varying health disparities that exist among all LGBTQ populations, both in the industrialized countries and in the global South. Some of this work will require advocacy to ensure that sexual identity questions are made part of standard surveillance efforts, so that we can not only replicate the findings of exploratory studies on a specific health disparity but also be in a position to identify the health disparities that create the greatest threat to morbidity and mortality among sexual minority populations. Research to identify the driving forces that create these health disparities will inspire the design of interventions and thus pave the way for eventual rigorous testing of interventions. Once efficacy of the interventions is measured and shows promise to reduce a pressing health disparity, work to bring the intervention to scale as part of public health practice can begin. The fact that this work must be undertaken on a global basis makes the agenda one of astonishing complexity and almost unparalleled excitement.

It should now be clear to readers why we decided to end this section of the book as a love note to future generations of researchers in LGBTQ health. A public health agenda that is this ambitious must include efforts to mentor future generations of researchers, who will build on the contributions made by the generations that preceded them. Emerging generations of researchers will make exciting contributions, of which we can now only dream, to understanding and resolving health disparities in LGBTQ populations. These contributions will allow LGBTQ communities to reinvest resources on other issues beyond fighting health disparities, which is likely to add to cultural vibrancy and increase the contributions of LGBTQ people to the larger society. We suspect that future contributions of LGBTQ health research will have many important repercussions for broader populations, since these contributions are based on the assumption that all members of a society should have equal access to health care. We can also hope and expect that models of health care delivery that are developed to raise levels of health in LGBTQ communities will provide important insights to efforts to resolve health disparities in other stigmatized communities.

Those who make contributions to ending health disparities among LGBTQ populations have thus chosen to work in an expanding area of science in which many new and important discoveries and contributions are possible. This work will be informed by a strong commitment to social justice and may well have a global reach. It will take on the difficult issue of translating biomedical and behavioral interventions into settings where work with stigmatized populations may not be welcome; if it succeeds, it will provide an important example for work with other marginalized populations. Thus, the investigators to whom our note is addressed are motivated by intellectual daring and a strong commitment to social justice and are willing to act in the real world based on the courage of their convictions. We hope that you will be able to use the research tools described in this book to further advance the field, and in so doing, make the world a better place.

PART 2 DESCRIPTIVE RESEARCH METHODS

Why Are Methods and Approaches So Important for LGBTQ Health Research?

Brian Dodge and Mark L. Hatzenbuehler

THE PLANS and procedures for research on sexual and gender minority (SGM) individuals, as well as the specific research methods of data collection, analysis, and interpretation, are of utmost importance in conducting and understanding research on LGBTQ, and other SGM individuals of diverse sexual and gender identities.[1,2] The health concerns and needs of LGBTQ individuals have been found to differ substantially from those of heterosexual individuals. Studies have consistently demonstrated that LGBTQ individuals tend to report poorer health outcomes relative to heterosexual individuals, including physical, mental, psychosocial, and sexual health.[1,3–5] We currently lack a comprehensive understanding of the causes of such disparities, particularly at the intersection of racial/ethnic and other identities, due to a relative lack of refined data on diverse SGM individuals. Public health researchers sometimes rely on categories based on sexual behavior (including MSM, men who have sex with men) for research that focuses on sexual risk and adverse sexual health outcomes (e.g., STI/HIV). This practice emerged from the early days of the HIV epidemic, when researchers rapidly learned that not all men who engage in sexual behavior with other men identify as "gay" or "bisexual." However, using behavioral categories interchangeably with sexual self-identity categories obfuscates the role that sexual identity may play in relation to health outcomes. And, on the other hand, using sexual identity as a selection criterion may be challenging, as some individuals are not "fixed" in terms of their sexual identities and may shift labels over time.[6,7] Thus, defining who and what constitutes the "LGBTQ population" (whether such a uniform population even exists) is in and of itself complex.

Who we are referring to in relation to LGBTQ health matters? In terms of sexual identity, much previous research focusing on self-identified lesbian, gay, and bisexual individuals has lumped together participants together in a monolithic category ("LGB") without examining differences between these groups based on identity.[8,9] (In terms of gender identity, transgender and other gender minority individuals are sometimes included in these studies—and oftentimes not.) This has resulted in limitations in our understanding of diverse groups who fall under the broad SGM umbrella. For example, collapsing bisexual and homosexual individuals under the common rubric of *LGB* has proved problematic in previous research. Research on bisexual men and women has illuminated numerous and profound differences in physical, mental, sexual, and other health outcomes when compared with exclusively homosexual *and* heterosexual men and women, including psychosocial health issues, such as depression, anxiety, substance use, violence victimization, and suicidality; health-risk behavior issues, such as unprotected sex, sex-work engagement, higher number of sexual partners, frequent use of emergency contraception and pregnancy termination; and biomedical health issues, including disproportionate rates of HIV and other STI, as well as lower health-related quality of life.[10–12] Researchers have recently posited that these differences are due, in part, to the unique "double discrimination" experienced by bisexual individuals from both straight and gay/lesbian individuals.

How, when, and where we access our research participants also matters. Researchers have characterized sampling as "the single most influential component of conducting research with lesbian, gay, and bisexual (LGB) populations."[2] This is certainly true of transgender and other gender minority populations, who are even more understudied than LGB populations, as well. The vast majority of early studies on health among LGBTQ individuals have been based on nonprobability convenience samples. Convenience sampling can result in skewed results that will mislead other researchers, policymakers, and practitioners. Following the above example, bisexual individuals are unlikely to be captured in traditional "gay-identified" venues, as they have been found to face stigma from both heterosexual and homosexual counterparts.[11, 13–16] Thus, a sample of "gay and bisexual women" recruited from gay community venues (e.g., bars, pride parades, etc.) is reflective only of the bisexual women who feel comfort and belonging within such settings.

Researchers who study sexual and gender minority populations have therefore recently devoted significant energy and resources to selecting research approaches based on plans that more comprehensively characterize the diversity of these individuals within the general US population. Such work is neither easy nor inexpensive. In addition to cost, a variety of issues historically prevented researchers from obtaining probability samples of LGBTQ individuals, including feasibility as well as social stigma surrounding homosexuality, bisexuality, and gender minorities.[17] As attitudes and norms have slowly become more tolerant in recent decades, with major social changes such as the recognition of same-sex marriages at a national level, researchers are now able to include sexual identity as a demographic characteristic (similar to gender, age, and race/ethnicity) on a scope that was not feasible in prior eras, thereby creating possibilities for constructing nationally representative sampling frames of sexual minority individuals.[18] In particular, recent technological innovations have facilitated the possibility of collecting data from samples of self-identified lesbian, gay, bisexual, and even other-identified (queer, pansexual, asexual) individuals in the United States that are probabilistic and reflective of a national-level population.[19,20] Still, we lack the ability to employ such techniques with transgender, nonbinary and other gender minority populations due largely to the fact that we have sparse even basic prevalence data on their numbers within the general population. Few national studies ask about gender identity, and even the Behavioral Risk Factor Surveillance System (BRFSS) gender identity module is optional and used by a small number of states.[21] Few other national studies ask about gender identity. In short, we have come a long way in terms of LGBTQ health but we still have a long way to go—and the methods and approaches we use matter.

In this part of the book, we provide an overview of a wide range of practical and theoretical considerations you will face when conducting research on health among sexual and gender minority issues, as well as best practices (and future recommendations) for doing this work. This section is broken up into five separate chapters that cover specific issues related to research methods and approaches with LGBTQ populations:

Chapter 4. *Definitions: "Straight, that is not gay"—Moving beyond Binary Notions of Sexual and Gender Identities* (Randall Sell and Kerith Conron)

Chapter 5. *Sampling Considerations for LGBTQ Health Research* (Christopher Owens, Ron Stall, and Brian Dodge)

Chapter 6. *Theory as a Practical Tool in Research and Intervention* (Ilan H. Meyer)

Chapter 7. *Creating and Adapting LGBTQ-Specific Measures to Explain Disparities* (Joshua G. Rosenberger)

Chapter 8. *Multilevel Approaches to Understanding LGBTQ Health Disparities* (Mark L. Hatzenbuehler)

Following these chapters, we introduce some of the unique "who, what, when, where, and why?" questions that LGBTQ health researchers strive to answer in their research. We also hope to also spark new questions for you to raise and explore in your own future research.

References
1. Institute of Medicine Committee on Lesbian Gay, Bisexual, and Transgender Health Issues and Research Gaps and Opportunities. *The Health of Lesbian, Gay, Bisexual, and Transgender People: Building a Foundation for Better Understanding.* Washington, DC: National Academies Press; 2011. Available from http://www.ncbi .nlm.nih.gov/books/NBK64806/.

2. Meyer, I. H., and Wilson, P. A. 2009. Sampling lesbian, gay, and bisexual populations. *Journal of Counseling Psychology* 56(1): 23–31.

3. Mayer K. H., Bradford, J. B., Makadon, H. J., Stall, R., Goldhammer, H., and Landers, S. 2008. Sexual and gender minority health: What we know and what needs to be done. *American Journal of Public Health* 98(6): 989–95.

4. Bostwick W. B., Boyd, C. J., Hughes, T. L., West, B. T., McCabe, S. E. 2014. Discrimination and mental health among lesbian, gay, and bisexual adults in the United States. *American Journal of Orthopsychiatry* 84(1): 35–45.

5. Wolitski, R., and Fenton, K. 2011. Sexual health, HIV, and sexually transmitted infections among gay, bisexual, and other men who have sex with men in the United States. *AIDS and Behavior* 15(1): 9–17.

6. Diamond, L. M. 2003. Was it a phase? Young women's relinquishment of lesbian/bisexual identities over a five-year period. *Journal of Personality and Social Psychology* 84(2): 352–64.

7. Savin-Williams, R.C., and Cohen, K. M. 2015. Developmental trajectories and milestones of lesbian, gay, and bisexual young people. *International Review of Psychiatry* 27(5): 357–66.

8. Dodge, B., Schnarrs, P., Reece, M., Martinez, O., Goncalves, G., Malebranche, D., Pol, B., Nix, R., and Fortenberry, J. 2013. Sexual behaviors and experiences among behaviorally bisexual men in the midwestern United States. *Archives of Sexual Behavior* 42(2): 247–56.

9. Sandfort, T. G. M., and Dodge, B. 2009. Homosexual and bisexual labels and behaviors among men: The need for clear conceptualizations, accurate operationalizations, and appropriate methodological designs. In V. Reddy, T. G. M. Sandfort, and R. Rispel eds., *Perspectives on Same-Sex Sexuality, Gender and HIV/AIDS in South Africa: From Social Silence to Social Science*, 51–57. Pretoria: Human Sciences Research Council.

10. Jeffries, W. L., IV. 2014. Beyond the bisexual bridge: Sexual health among U.S. men who have sex with men and women. *American Journal of Preventive Medicine* 47(3): 320–29.

11. Friedman, M. R., Dodge, B., Schick, V., Herbenick, D., Hubach, R., Bowling, J., Goncalves, G., Krier, S., and Reece, M. 2014. From bias to bisexual health disparities: Attitudes toward bisexual men and women in the United States. *LGBT Health* 1(4): 309–18.

12. Mereish E. H., Katz-Wise, S. L., and Woulfe, J. 2017. Bisexual-specific minority stressors, psychological distress, and suicidality in bisexual individuals: The mediating role of loneliness. *Prevention Science* 18(6): 716–25.

13. Dodge, B., Schnarrs, P. W., Reece, M., Goncalves, G., Martinez, O., Nix, R., Malebranche, D., Van Der Pol, B., Murray, M., Fortenberry, J. D. 2012. Community involvement among behaviourally bisexual men in the Midwestern USA: Experiences and perceptions across communities. *Culture, Health & Sexuality* 14(9): 1095–110.

14. Dodge, B., and Sandfort, T. G. M.2007 A review of mental health research on bisexual individuals when compared to homosexual and heterosexual individuals. In B. A. Firestein, ed., *Becoming Visible: Counseling Bisexuals across the Lifespan*, 28–51. New York: Columbia University Press.

15. Herek, G. M. 2002. Heterosexuals' attitudes toward bisexual men and women in the United States. *Journal of Sex Research* 39(4): 264–74.

16. Yost M., and Thomas, G. 2012. Gender and binegativity: Men's and women's attitudes toward male and female bisexuals. *Archives of Sexual Behavior* 41(3): 691–702.

17. Sell, R. L., and Holliday, M. L. 2014. Sexual orientation data collection policy in the United States: Public health malpractice. *American Journal of Public Health* 104(6): 967–69.

18. Hays, R., Liu, H., and Kapteyn, A. 2015. Use of Internet panels to conduct surveys. *Behavior Research Methods* 47(3): 685–90.

19. Dodge, B., Herbenick, D., Friedman, M. R., Schick, V., Fu, T. J., Bostwick, W., Bartelt, E., Muñoz-Laboy, M., Pletta, D. Reece, M., and Sandfort, T. G. 2016. Attitudes toward bisexual men and women among a nationally representative probability sample of adults in the United States. *PloS One* 11(10): e0164430.

20. Dodge, B., Herbenick, D., Fu, T. C., Schick, V., Reece, M., Sanders, S., and Fortenberry, J. D. 2016. Sexual behaviors of U.S. men by self-identified sxual orientation: Results from the 2012 National Survey of Sexual Health and Behavior. *Journal of Sexual Medicine* 13(4): 637–49.

21. Centers for Medicare & Medicaid Services. 2019. *Behavioral Risk Factor Surveillance System (BRFSS). Sexual and Gender Minority Clearinghouse.* https://www.cms.gov/About-CMS/Agency-Information/OMH/resource-center/hcps-and-researchers/data-tools/sgm-clearinghouse/brfss.html.

FOUR

Definitions: "Straight, that is not gay"

Moving beyond Binary Notions of Sexual
and Gender Identities

Randall Sell and Kerith Conron

BEFORE DESCRIBING the health of a population, or for that matter anything else about them, a researcher needs to delineate the population. Delineating the population is a two-step process. The first step is *defining the population*; the second is identifying a process for *categorizing individuals* as members of the population (or as *not* members of the population). For the most part, all populations are socially constructed (e.g., by race, ethnicity, or religion), and their complex histories must be understood before undertaking any research on any group.[1,2] For example, it is negligent to study gay men without first describing what you mean by *gay* and *men*, and it is only possible to compare two studies describing gay men if each has used the same definitions and measures to guide its research. Additionally, it is a major flaw to collapse *gay* and *bisexual men* into an arbitrary, monolithic category without acknowledging the vast literature demonstrating that bisexual individuals report higher rates of nearly all negative health outcomes (including depression, anxiety, eating disorders, substance abuse, suicidality, and sexual health concerns) as well as structural inequities (including poverty, lack of access to healthcare, and lack of tailored health intervention programs) when compared with both heterosexual and gay/

lesbian individuals. Put more simply, even if you *say* you are comparing apples to apples, are you *really* comparing apples to apples, or are you comparing apples to oranges? Unfortunately, few researchers give as much critical thought to population definition and measurement as they should; many give no thought at all to this topic, as evidenced by the state of published research.

If we were to design a research study *today,* we would use the following question to assess the sexual orientation of potential research subjects:

> *Sexual Orientation:* Which of the following best represents how you think of yourself? Gay or Lesbian, Straight, that is not gay, Bisexual, Something else, I don't know.[3]

Other researchers might use different terminology, as discussed elsewhere in this book; see "The Challenges of Language," page 13. And we would use the following questions to assess gender identity and sex and to facilitate, on the basis of these two questions, the identification of individuals that are transgender or cisgender:

> *Gender Identity:* What is your current gender identity? Male, Female, Transgender, Genderqueer/Gender non-conforming, I am not sure of my gender identity, I don't know what this question is asking.

> *Sex:* What sex were you assigned at birth, on your original birth certificate? Male, Female.

We want to emphasize that these are the questions we would use as of the writing of this chapter. These are not the questions that we would have recommended even a few months ago, and we cannot imagine that they will be the questions we recommend a few years from now. So if you want to conduct up-to-date research on sexual and gender minorities, then you are going to need to do some critical thinking and additional review of recent literature on your own. Moreover, you should feel free to disagree with our recommendation of these questions, but such disagreements should be founded on more than opinion and ideally on findings from empirical investigations. These questions are based on our current fundamental understanding of the constructs of sexual orientation, gender identity, and sex, and they reflect which questions we believe are best able to sort people into categories. The process of moving from definitions of abstract populations to the creation of tangible measures to assess these definitions, while recognizing the constantly shifting sand on which you are building these measures, is difficult at best.

Some researchers have argued that the necessarily constant process of updating definitions and measures to reflect shifting social constructs is futile. And some academics have argued that the imperfect process allows only for the further reification of categories that have limited social value.[4,5] By putting people into boxes and labeling them *bisexual* or *transgender*, are we causing them further harm? Counter to these concerns, we would argue that sexual and gender minorities are being harmed socially and politically, and without research to understand these injuries, we only allow them to persist. We believe that data provide power to understand issues and disparities that can then be addressed through social programs and policies, but we also recognize that data can be used to harm and to further amplify disparities. On the whole, however, we trust that the positive value of data far outweighs any potential negative effects.

Below we provide a basic introduction to these issues, presenting a brief review of the social construction and definition of sexual and gender minorities followed by a brief introduction to the history of the measurement of sexual orientation, gender identity, and sex.

LGBTQ Measurement Research from the Birth of the LGBTQ Health Movement until the Present

To adequately measure a phenomenon of interest, one must first clearly define that phenomenon. At this stage in LGBTQ health research, increasingly referred to as research on sexual orientation and gender identity (SOGI), sexual orientation is commonly defined as a multidimensional construct that consists of at least three primary dimensions: attraction, behavior, and identity.[6] Due to significant advocacy starting in the late 1990s,[7] and measurement development and assessment research, much of it conducted by members of the Sexual Minority Assessment Research Team (SMART)[8–10] between 2000 and 2008, several measures of each dimension of sexual orientation have been formulated and used in an array of surveys.[11] At this point, the refinement and assessment of sexual orientation measures, particularly in languages other than English, and for specific population subgroups (older adults, transgender people, non-US-born individuals), are priorities for the advancement of population-based sexual orientation data collection.

Advocacy around inclusion of survey measures that would make the needs of transgender respondents visible began to emerge around the turn of the millennium—propelled by findings from HIV needs-assessment studies of transgender women in urban areas around the United States.[12–16] Importantly, the expertise of transgender community organizers and providers informed these needs assessments and provided opportunities for discussion about how and what to measure in matters related to sex and gender identity. Measurement research on gender identity, assigned sex at birth, and related constructs (e.g., transgender status, gender expression), did not gain significant momentum for another five to ten years.[17–24] Advocacy and measurement research related to sex and gender for use in public health settings accelerated in 2011,[17,18] propelled by the release of findings from the National Survey on Transgender Experiences of Discrimination in the United States,[25] and following two invited meetings on transgender-inclusive health surveillance convened by Health and Human Services Secretary Kathleen Sebelius. In 2011, former members of SMART and other colleagues at the Williams Institute of the UCLA School of Law formed a multidisciplinary group of experts to develop population-based data about transgender people and other gender minorities. Between 2011 and 2013, the Gender Identity in US Surveillance (GenIUSS) group reviewed current practices to identify transgender and other gender minority respondents in population research, conducted two studies to address gaps in knowledge about measure performance, and made policy recommendations regarding measurement research and data collection.

In September 2014, GenIUSS released a report summarizing its efforts titled *Best Practices for Asking Questions to Identify Transgender and Other Gender Minority Respondents on Population-Based Surveys.*[26] Much of the material on gender identity and sex for this chapter was contributed by Kerith Conron for the GenIUSS Best Practices Report. Thus, definitions of core constructs and recommendations for measures of sex and gender identity contained in this chapter reflect consensus among a group of scientists, advocates, scholars, and community members at a recent point in time, with the expectation that measures will be refined with further testing and that they will change over time as the phenomena themselves (especially gender identity) evolve.

Defining the Populations
Sexual Orientation

Over the previous century and a half, many different terms and definitions have been used to describe sexual orientations.[27] Karl Heinrich Ulrichs proposed one of the earliest and most important classification schemes of the sexual orientation construct. In a series of pamphlets published in German in the 1860s (and formally translated into English only well over a century later), he separated males into three basic categories: *Dionings, Urnings,* and *Uranodionings* (table 4.1).[28] These terms were derived from a speech by Pausanias in Plato's *Symposium* in which Pausanias associates the love of men for other males with Aphrodite Urania (the daughter of Uranus); love for females is associated with Aphrodite Paneumia (the daughter of Zeus and Dione). The categories as described by Ulrichs objectively correspond to the predominant categories used today: heterosexual, homosexual, and bisexual. Ulrichs referred to women, whose sexual orientations were largely ignored in the writings of early researchers, as *Urningins* if they were homosexual; heterosexual women were referred to as *Dioningins.*[28]

Xavier Mayne, who followed Ulrichs and was influenced by his works, provided a formal definition of an Urning in the first major work on homosexuality to be written by an American: "a human being that is more or less perfectly, even distinctly, masculine in physique; often a virile type of fine intellectual, oral and aesthetic sensibilities: but who, through an inborn or later-developed preference feels sexual passion for

Table 4.1 Karl Ulrich's Male Sexual Orientation Taxonomy

Ulrich's Taxonomy	Gender Characteristics
Dioning	Comparable to the modern term *heterosexual*. A Dioning who behaves like an Urning is termed a *Uraniaster*.
Urning	Comparable to the modern term *homosexual*
Mannling	A manly Urning
Weibling	An effeminate Urning
Zwischen	A somewhat manly and somewhat effeminate Urning
Virilisiert	An Urning who behaves sexually like a Dioning
Urano-Dioning	Comparable to the modern term *bisexual*

Source: Adapted from http://www.lgbtdata.com/karl-ulrichs-sexual-orientation-classification-scheme.html. For additional information, see K. H. Ulrichs, *The Riddle of Manly Love* (Buffalo, NY: Prometheus Books, 1994); and E. Carpenter, *The Intermediate Sex* (London: Allen and Unwin, 1908).

the male human species. His sexual preference may quite exclude any desire for the female sex; or may exist concurrently with that instinct."[29] Mayne's definition overlaps with Ulrichs's male Uranodionings by stating that desire for the female sex may exist concurrently.

Ulrichs's writings influenced the works of many other early researchers, including Westphal, Richard von Krafft-Ebing, Albert Moll, Edward Carpenter, Havelock Ellis, John Addington Symonds, and Magnus Hirschfeld.[30–37] Through the works of these writers and researchers, Ulrichs should be credited with influencing almost every attempt to describe sexual minorities to the present day, albeit indirectly. Even the terms *homosexuality* and *heterosexuality* are linked directly to him, though Ulrichs preferred his own terminology. They first appeared in a letter to Ulrichs dated May 6, 1868, from Karl-Maria Benkert, a German-Hungarian physician and writer.[28] In a pamphlet published in 1869. Benkert provided the following definition of homosexuality:

> In addition to the normal sexual urge in man and woman, Nature in her sovereign mood has endowed at birth certain male and female individuals with the homosexual urge, thus placing them in a sexual bondage which renders them physically and psychically incapable—even with the best intention—of normal erection. This urge creates in advance a direct horror of the opposite sexual [sic] and the victim of this passion finds it impossible to suppress the feeling which individuals of his own sex exercise upon him.[38]

As the term *homosexuality* (from the Greek word *homos,* meaning "same" and the Latin word *sexus,* meaning "sex") and later *heterosexuality* gained currency, many writers and researchers deemed its mixture of Greek and Latin inappropriate, but attempts to replace the terms were futile; they were too deeply rooted in the literature by the time Greek and Latin purists arrived on the scene. It is believed that the term *homosexual* was first introduced into English by Symonds in his first edition of *A Problem of Modern Ethics*, which he published privately in England in 1891, but the term appeared in 1892 in the more widely distributed English translation of Krafft-Ebing's *Psychopathia Sexualis.*[39]

Sexual orientations are most commonly described today using the terms *heterosexual* (straight), *homosexual* (gay and lesbian), and *bisexual.*[40] Because researchers and writers have focused more on homosexuality than on heterosexuality or bisexuality, many more terms have evolved to describe homosexuality, including uranianism, homogenic love, contrasexuality, homoerotism, similsexualism, tribadism, sexual inversion, intersexuality, transexuality, third sex, and psychosexual hermaphroditism.[28,30,35,41] Even over the past several decades, we have seen a shifting terminology as the word *homosexual* becomes less acceptable than the terms *gay* or *lesbian*, and the word *heterosexual*, which never gained widespread popular use, is less preferable to the word *straight*. And terms that once were considered offensive have become less so. For example, the term *queer* was defined by Gershon Legman in 1941 as: "Homosexual; more often used of male homosexuals than of Lesbians. As an adjective it is the most common in use in America."[42] At the time Legman wrote, the term was slang and used primarily, but not exclusively, pejoratively. In current usage, the term still primarily refers to lesbians and gays, but it is frequently used nonpejoratively in scholarly works and within sexual and gender minority communities.[43-45] For some, *queer* has come to serve as an umbrella term that includes all lesbian, gay, bisexual, and transgender people.

When researchers and writers refer to sexual minorities, they are usually speaking about people with sexual orientations other than the majority (i.e., heterosexual/straight). However, the broader construct, sexual orientation, itself has a wide variety of definitions and meanings.

These definitions generally include one or both of two components: one generally uses "psychological" language, and the other uses "behavioral" language. Mayne's definition of the term *Urning* and Benkert's definition of the term *homosexual*, which are the earliest definitions available, interestingly describe only the psychological (not behavioral) state. Mayne's definition alludes to how feelings of sexual passion govern an individual's sexual orientation, while Benkert writes about an "urge."[29,38]

Ellis, perhaps the most important and influential writer on sexual orientation in late nineteenth- and early twentieth-century England, also included a purely psychological component in his definition of homosexuality as a "sexual instinct turned by inborn constitutional abnormality toward persons of the same sex."[46] Ellis used the term *sexual inversion* at the time this definition was formulated, but in later versions of his work he substituted the term *homosexuality*. Similarly, excluding any discussion of behavioral aspects, the first two medical journal articles about homosexuality to appear in the English language include a translation of Westphal's German definition, which describes homosexuals as persons who "as a result of their inborn nature felt themselves drawn by sexual desire to male individuals exclusively."[47,48]

These early definitions are of interest because they almost uniformly exclude any behavioral component (and in particular behavior that is sexual), except to describe the thought of sexual behavior with the other sex as "repulsive" or "horrifying" to the homosexual. For example, Auguste Forel (1924) in his popular book *The Sexual Question*, states:

> However shocking or absurd the aberrations of the sexual appetite and its irradiations may be, of which we have spoken hitherto, they are at any rate derived from originally normal intercourse with adults of the opposite sex. Those we have now to deal with are distinguished by the fact that not only the appetite itself, but all its psychic irradiations are directed to the same sex as the perverted individual, the latter being horrified at the idea of genital contact with the opposite sex, quite as much as a normal man is horrified at the idea of homosexual union.[49]

Krafft-Ebing, like his contemporaries, even went so far as to exclude behavior from the diagnosis of homosexuality. In *Psychopathia Sexualis*, he states that "the determining factor here is the demonstration of perverse feelings for the same sex; not the proof of sexual acts with the same sex. These two phenomena must not be confounded with each other."[34]

More recent definitions often include both psychological and behavioral components. Simon LeVay, for example, defined sexual orientation as "the direction of sexual feelings or behavior, toward individuals of the opposite sex (heterosexuality), the same sex (homosexuality), or some combination of the two (bisexuality)," and James D. Weinrich defined homosexuality "either (1) as a genital act or (2) as a long-term sexuoerotic status."[50–52] Here the psychological states referred to are "sexual feelings" and "sexuoerotic status," and the behavioral outcome, as referred to by LeVay and Weinrich is "sexual behavior" and a "genital act" respectively. What is further interesting and complicating in these definitions is that the two components in both definitions are connected by "or," which indicates that either can be used to assess sexual orientation.

Other definitions include both psychological and behavioral components, joined by the conjunction "and." For example, *A Descriptive Dictionary and Atlas of Sexology* describes homosexuality as "the occurrence or existence of sexual attraction, interest and genitally intimate activity between an individual and other members of the same gender."[53] Here there are two psychological components, "sexual attraction" and "interest," and one behavioral component, which is described as "genitally intimate activity." The presence of the conjunction "and" makes it difficult to interpret whether both components are necessary for the classification of sexual orientations. And while most definitions include some psychological component, some descriptions of sexual orientation allude only to a behavioral component. For example, in 1973 *Stedman's Medical Dictionary* defined homosexuality as "sexual behavior, including sexual congress, between individuals of the same sex, especially past puberty."[54]

Frank Beach goes so far as to state that when discussing homosexuality he is referring only to same-sex sexual behavior. In his introduction to the first English language translation of André Gide's defense of homosexuality, *Corydon*, Beach states: "The term [homosexuality] means different things to different people . . . it is preferable to set forth the significance of the term as used in this discussion. Homosexuality refers exclusively to overt behavior between two individuals of the same sex. The behavior must be patently sexual, involving erotic arousal and, in most instances at least, resulting in the satisfaction of the sexual urge."[55]

Further complicating this discussion is that the psychological and behavioral components of the definitions of sexual orientation discussed thus far are not uniform, but rather vary in significant and conflicting ways. Psychological components of definitions include the terms *sexual desire, sexual passion, sexual feelings, sexual urge, sexual attraction, sexual interest, sexual arousal, affectional preference, sexual instinct, sexual orientation identity,* and *sexual preference.* In some instances, *sexual preference* has been used in place of the term *sexual orientation,* but numerous writers have indicated that they believe it is misleading because the word *preference* implies the capacity to choose to whom you are attracted.[56] We recommend using the label *sexual orientation* rather than *sexual preference* for the construct because research indicates that same-sex and/or opposite-sex sexual feelings are for most people a basic established part of an individual's awareness significantly earlier than conscious choice would indicate. Finally, it is important to note that each of these descriptions, even when they use the same words, may have a distinct meaning in the context that they are used, and are not necessarily indicative of the same phenomenon when different writers use them. That is, different terms in definitions may be describing slightly different phenomena despite the use of the same label to describe those phenomena.

The behavioral components of these definitions show dramatic but equally important variations. Some of the behavioral components we have come across have been described as *sexual behavior, genital activity, sexual intercourse, sexual contact,* or *sexual contact that achieves orgasm.* Each of these presents further challenges for researchers in that they further require definition. For example, the definition of *sexual intercourse* varies dramatically, often involving very intimate discussions of sexual behavior.

The variations among these definitions and terms cannot be fully reviewed here, but we hope we have provided a broad overview of some of the important issues that need to be considered when conducting research. While it is not possible from this review to say that one definition or set of terms is "better" than another, we recommend that researchers who collect sexual orientation data explicitly define the terms they use to describe populations when presenting research results. That way, consumers of the research can compare the findings with other studies and determine whether they are comparing apples to apples, or apples to oranges.

Gender Identity and Sex

Although discourse on the distinction between sex and gender emerged in the public health literature in 2003, via a seminal paper by Nancy Krieger,[57] recent[58] and current work often attempts to push for a clear articulation of the underlying phenomenon—the cornerstone of measurement research. While the terms *gender* and *sex* are often used interchangeably, in both scientific contexts[59,60] and in lay usage,[21] they reflect different constructs and should be assessed with different measures. *Gender* is a multidimensional, time-varying construct that includes identity and expression (e.g., as masculine or feminine through appearance and behavior),[61] while the term *sex* is generally used to refer to biological differences (hormones, secondary sex characteristics, reproductive anatomy).[57] Although sex is commonly described as a fixed or static trait in many epidemiological contexts, sex is also multidimensional and can be altered over time through the use of hormones and surgical intervention. Assigned sex at birth—the sex recorded on the birth certificate by medical practitioners, typically based on the appearance of external genitalia—is often of primary interest in public health. It is important to note that assigned sex at birth (as recorded on the original birth certificate) serves as the basis for sex as legally construed; sex can sometimes be changed on legal documents (i.e., driver's license, passport, birth certificate) through a complex set of procedures.

Cisgender (nontransgender) individuals can be identified through consistent responses to questions about assigned sex at birth and current gender identity, while transgender individuals can be identified through inconsistent responses to the same questions. The term *gender identity* refers to an individual's internal sense of being a male or female, genderqueer, and so forth and may reflect an affiliation with a particular community (e.g., women, transmen, transgender.) *Transgender* is a term used to describe a diverse group of individuals whose current gender identity and/or expression is not fully congruent with their assigned sex at birth.[62,63] Importantly, as described below, some individuals classified as transgender may identity their gender identity as transgender, but many others do not.

Categorizing Individuals

Researchers have attempted to devise measures (usually one or more questions) to categorize individuals into groups, ideally on the basis of sound reasoning and definitions such as those discussed above. Below we outline some of the measures that have been used to assess sexual orientation, gender identity, and sex.

Sexual Orientation

Ulrichs, in a series of pamphlets published in the 1860s, outlined a sequence of questions that could be asked to determine whether a man was an Urning.[28] These questions, translated from the German, included the following:

1. Does he feel for males and only for males a passionate yearning of love, be it gushing and gentle, or fiery and sensual?
2. Does he feel horror at sexual contact with women? This horror may not always be found but when it is found, it is decisive.
3. Does he experience a beneficial magnetic current when making contact with a male body in its prime?
4. Does the excitement of attraction find its apex in the male sexual organs?

Mayne, who was a follower of Ulrichs, went even further, outlining a series of several hundred questions for the classification of Urnings and Urningins.[29] These questions include the following:

1. At what age did your sexual desire show itself distinctly?
2. Did it direct itself at first most to the male or to the female sex? Or did it hesitate awhile between both?

3. Is the instinct unvaryingly toward the male or female sex now? Or do you take pleasure (or would you experience it) with now a man, now a woman?

. 4. Do you give way to it rather mentally or physically? Or are both in equal measure?

5. Is the similsexual desire constant, periodic or irregularly felt?

6. In dreams, do you have visions of sexual relations with men or women, the more frequently and ardently?

The respondents were expected to be able to provide yes-or-no answers to the series of questions outlined by Ulrichs and Mayne, which allowed them to be classified as an *Urning*, or *Urningin*, or neither. Simple yes-or-no classifications of sexual orientation have historically been simplified, with subjects usually classified as homosexual or not homosexual (usually labeled straight or heterosexual), with a third category "bisexual" the most significant difference from the earliest classification schemes. In major health surveys, we would argue that the state-of-the-art question to assess sexual orientations, which is an example of the simplest type of measure, is:

Which of the following best represents how you think of yourself? Gay or Lesbian; Straight: that is not gay; Bisexual; Something else; I don't know.

Again, other researchers may use different items to assess sexual orientation.

This question was designed and tested for use on the National Health Interview Survey (NHIS).[3] A number of things should be noted about this question. First, the stem of the question asks "how you think of yourself" rather than asking about the individual's sexual orientation because many people do not know what the term *sexual orientation* means. It is from the array of possible responses to the question that respondents figure out what the question is about. Second, the question puts the response category "gay or lesbian" first so that straight people will know that that category has already been asked and that the category that fits them should be coming soon. The second response, "straight, that is not gay" helps straight people figure out which category to pick by indicating that *straight* is *not gay* (which assumes that the two are mutually exclusive; that is not always the case!). The third response is "bisexual," which comes with its own inherent complexities (with an increasing number of researchers using the term "bisexual+" to include other fluid sexual identities including pansexual, queer, as well as those who do not adhere to fixed identity labels. The fourth response category, "I don't know," should not be interpreted as implying that the respondent does not know their sexual orientation, but more likely that they don't understand the question.

Despite the focus on single-question measures in most surveys conducted today, more sophisticated measures of sexual orientation have been proposed; several of the more important ones are reviewed here. Of these, perhaps the most important is the Kinsey scale, which Alfred Kinsey used to study people in his famous books on the human male and human female.[41,64] Kinsey et al. proposed a bipolar scale that allows for a continuum between "exclusive heterosexuality," which is labeled 0, and "exclusive homosexuality," which is labeled 6 (table 4.2). Exclusively homosexual individuals became known colloquially as *Kinsey 6*s. Kinsey et al. were the first to recognize the continuous nature of sexual orientation, and their measure departed dramatically from the dichotomous measures of those that came before. Kinsey provided the following rationales for this decision:

> The world is not to be divided into sheep and goats. Not all things are black nor all things white. It is a fundamental of taxonomy that nature rarely deals with discrete categories. Only the human mind invents categories and tries to force facts into separated pigeon-holes. The living world is a continuum in each and every one of its aspects. The sooner we learn this concerning human sexual behavior the sooner we shall reach a sound understanding of the realities of sex.[41] It is characteristic of the human mind that it tries to dichotomize in its classification of phenomena. Things are either so, or they are not so. Sexual behavior is either normal or abnormal, socially acceptable or unacceptable, heterosexual or homosexual; and many persons do not want to believe that there are gradations in these matters from one to the other extreme.[64]

Table 4.2 The Kinsey Scale

Rating	Description	Orientation
0	Exclusively heterosexual	Individuals who make no physical contacts with individuals of their own sex that result in erotic arousal or orgasm, and make no psychic responses to individuals of their own sex
1	Predominantly heterosexual/only incidentally homosexual	Individuals who have only incidental homosexual contacts which have involved physical or psychic response, or incidental psychic response without physical contact
2	Predominantly heterosexual but more than incidentally homosexual	Individuals who have more than incidental homosexual experience, and/or if they respond rather definitely to homosexual stimuli
3	Equally heterosexual and homosexual	Individuals who are about equally homosexual and heterosexual in their overt experience and/or their psychic reactions
4	Predominantly homosexual but more than incidentally heterosexual	Individuals who have more overt activity and/or psychic reactions in the homosexual, while still maintaining a fair amount of heterosexual activity and/or responding rather definitive to heterosexual contact
5	Predominantly homosexual/only incidentally heterosexual	Individuals who are almost entirely homosexual in their overt activities and/or reactions
6	Exclusively homosexual	Individuals who are exclusively homosexual, both in regard to their overt experience and in regard to their psychic reactions

Source: Adapted from A. C. Kinsey, W. B. Pomeroy, and C. E. Martin, *Sexual Behavior in the Human Male* (Philadelphia: W.B. Saunders, 1948); A. C. Kinsey, W. B. Pomeroy, C. E., Martin, and P. H. Gebhard, *Sexual Behavior in the Human Female* (Philadelphia: W. B. Saunders, 1953).

By deviating from the dichotomous classifications that preceded him and developing a bipolar continuous model, Kinsey created a new way of measuring sexual orientation that provided a new perspective on sexuality. That said, the Kinsey measure still forces individuals into one of seven categories and is therefore not a true continuum, which soon became a challenge for researchers. William Masters and Virginia Johnson noted the difficulty of using the Kinsey scale in their major study of homosexuality:

There was also concern in arbitrarily selecting the specific classification of Kinsey grades 2 through 4 for any individual who had had a large number of both homosexual and heterosexual experiences. The ratings were assigned by the research team after detailed history-taking, but it is difficult for any individual to be fully objective in assessing the amount of his or her heterosexual versus homosexual experience when there has been a considerable amount of both types of interaction. Some of these preferences ratings might well be subject to different interpretation by other health-care professionals.[65]

Masters and Johnson further observed:

Kinsey 3 classification was the most difficult to assign of the ratings. Relative equality in any form of diverse physical activity is hard to establish. Particularly was this so when the interviewer, in attempting to separate mature sexual experience into its homosexual and heterosexual components, was faced with a history of a multiplicity of partners of either sex. The problem was augmented by the subjects' frequently vague recall of the average number of sexual interactions with each partner.[65]

A second concern with the Kinsey Scale, the researchers soon discovered, is that it sometimes classifies into the same categories individuals who are significantly different based upon specific aspects or dimensions of sexuality. In his own work, Kinsey used "overt sexual experience" and "psychosexual reactions," collected from the history of the subject in order to assign a category on his scale. In his first work, Kinsey alluded to the difficulties of using his scale: "It will be observed that the rating which an individual receives has a dual basis. It takes into account his overt sexual experience and/or his psychosexual reactions. In the majority of instances the two aspects of the history parallel but sometimes they are not in accord. In the latter case, the rating of an individual must be based upon an evaluation of the relative importance of the overt and the psychic in his history."[41]

Recognizing that valuable information was being lost by collapsing different dimensions of sexuality into a single score, researchers began to develop additional measures. The most obvious solution to avoid the loss of information was to assess dimensions of sexual orientation independently and report the scores separately. For example, Fritz Klein and colleagues proposed the Klein Sexual Orientation Grid (KSOG), which includes the assessment of seven dimensions of sexual orientation: sexual attraction, sexual behavior, sexual fantasies, emotional preference, social preference, self-identification, and heterosexual/homosexual lifestyle (table 4.3).[66] A significant problem with assessing multiple dimensions in a scale like the KSOG is that the results can be difficult for researchers to interpret, particularly when different dimensions do not perfectly correspond to each other. Consequently, researchers tend to limit the number of dimensions assessed, with sexual identity being the most commonly assessed.[67]

A third concern with the Kinsey Scale, some have argued, is that it inappropriately measures homosexuality and heterosexuality on the same scale, making one the trade-off of the other rather than recognizing them as independent constructs. This idea arose out of research in the 1970s on masculinity and femininity which found that the concepts of masculinity and femininity could, and perhaps should, be more appropriately measured independently.[68] Measuring them separately

Table 4.3 The Klein Sexual Orientation Grid

Variable	Past	Present	Ideal
A. Sexual attraction			
B. Sexual behavior			
C. Sexual fantasies			
D. Emotional preferences			
E. Social preferences			
F. Self-Identification			
G. Heterosexual/Homosexual lifestyle			

Notes

I. Scale to Measure Dimensions A, B, C, D, and E of the Klein Sexual Orientation Grid
0. Other sex only
1. Other sex mostly
2. Other sex somewhat
3. Both sexes equally

II. Scale to Measure Dimensions F and G of the Klein Sexual Orientation Grid
0. Heterosexual only
1. Heterosexual mostly
2. Heterosexual more
3. Heterosexual/homosexual equally

For additional information, see F. Klein, B. Sepekoff, and T. J. Wolf, Sexual orientation: A multi-variable dynamic process, *Journal of Homosexuality* 11 (1985): 35–49.

recognized masculinity and femininity as independent constructs rather than as separate ends of a continuum. When they were measured on the same scale, masculinity and femininity became trade-offs: to become more masculine, you had to be less feminine or vice versa. But measured separately, individuals could be very masculine *and* very feminine—or not very much of either, which previous bipolar measures would not allow. Measuring masculinity and femininity independently also allow for the identification of androgynous people on measures for the first time. Similarly, considering homosexuality and heterosexuality on separate scales allowed respondents to be very heterosexual and very homosexual (bisexual) at the same time, or not very much of either (asexual). V. L. Bullough discusses these issues in his following critique of the Kinsey scale: "I am, however, at this point in my research, convinced that the Kinsey scale has outlived its political usefulness and we need a more effective scholarly measuring tool. In fact, the Kinsey scale offers the same kind of difficulty that the traditional masculine-feminine scale did until it was realized that women could have masculine traits and still be feminine and vice versa."[69]

This idea of measuring homosexuality and heterosexuality separately was first put into practice by Michael Shively and John DeCecco, who created a five-point scale on which heterosexuality and homosexuality could be independently assessed (see fig 4.1).[70,71] Further, using this scale, in recognition of the multidimensional nature of sexual orientation, they proposed the assessment of two dimensions of sexual orientation: physical and affectional preference. While theoretically very interesting, Shively and DeCecco's scale was never widely used.

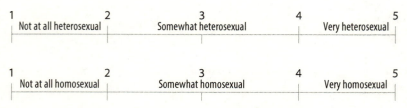

Figure 4.1. The Shively Scale of Sexual Orientation. After M. G. Shively and J. P. DeCecco, Components of sexual identity, *Journal of Homosexuality* 3 (1977): 41–48.

In recognition of all of the major concerns discussed above, the Sell Assessment of Sexual Orientation was created in the early 1990s.[72] To address these concerns, the Sell Assessment measures sexual orientation on a continuum (like Kinsey), considers different dimensions of sexual orientation (like KSOG), and considers homosexuality and heterosexuality separately (like Shively and DeCecco). The Sell Assessment contains twelve questions: six assess sexual attractions, four assess sexual behavior, and two assess sexual orientation identity. The Sell Assessment of Sexual Orientation was created to foster discussions about the measurement of sexual orientations, not necessarily to provide a definitive solution to the question of how to best measure this construct. In fact, the single identity question now in use on the NHIS is preferable for most research purposes.

The Sell Assessment of Sexual Orientation

I. Sexual Attractions

The following six questions are asked to assess how frequently and intensely you are sexually attracted to men and women. Consider times you had sexual fantasies, daydreams, or dreams about a man or woman, or have been sexually aroused by a man or woman.

1. During the *past year*, how many *different men* were you sexually attracted to (choose one answer):
   a. None
   b. 1
   c. 2
   d. 3–5
   e. 6–10
   f. 11–49
   g. 50–99
   h. 100 or more

2. During the *past year*, on average, how often were you sexually attracted to a *man* (choose one answer):
   a. Never
   b. Less than 1 time per month
   c. 1–3 times per month

(*continued*)

    d. 1 time per week

    e. 2–3 times per week

    f. 4–6 times per week

    g. Daily

3. During the *past year*, the most I was sexually attracted to a *man* was (choose one answer):
   a. Not at all sexually attracted
   b. Slightly sexually attracted
   c. Mildly sexually attracted
   d. Moderately sexually attracted
   e. Significantly sexually attracted
   f. Very sexually attracted
   g. Extremely sexually attracted

4. During the *past year*, how many *different women* were you sexually attracted to (choose one answer):
   a. None
   b. 1
   c. 2
   d. 3–5
   e. 6–10
   f. 11–49
   g. 50–99
   h. 100 or more

5. During the *past year*, on average, how often were you sexually attracted to a *woman* (choose one answer):
   a. Never
   b. Less than 1 time per month
   c. 1–3 times per month
   d. 1 time per week
   e. 2–3 times per week
   f. 4–6 times per week
   g. Daily

6. During the *past year*, the most I was sexually attracted to a *woman* was (choose one answer):
   a. Not at all sexually attracted
   b. Slightly sexually attracted
   c. Mildly sexually attracted

d. Moderately sexually attracted

e. Significantly sexually attracted

f. Very sexually attracted

g. Extremely sexually attracted

II. Sexual Contact

The following four questions are asked to assess your sexual contacts. Consider times when you had contact between your body and another man or woman's body for the purpose of sexual arousal or gratification.

7. During the *past year*, how many *different men* did you have sexual contact with (choose one answer):

   a. None

   b. 1

   c. 2

   d. 3–5

   e. 6–10

   f. 11–49

   g. 50–99

   h. 100 or more

8. During the *past year*, on average, how often did you have sexual contact with a *man* (choose one answer):

   a. Never

   b. Less than 1 time per month

   c. 1–3 times per month

   d. 1 time per week

   e. 2–3 times per week

   f. 4–6 times per week

   g. Daily

9. During the *past year*, how many *different women* did you have sexual contact with (choose one answer):

   a. None

   b. 1

   c. 2

   d. 3–5

   e. 6–10

   f. 11–49

(*continued*)

  g. 50–99

  h. 100 or more

10. During the *past year*, on average, how often did you have sexual contact with a woman (choose one answer):

  a. Never

  b. Less than 1 time per month

  c. 1–3 times per month

  d. 1 time per week

  e. 2–3 times per week

  f. 4–6 times per week

  g. Daily

III. Sexual Orientation Identity

The following two questions are asked to assess your sexual orientation identity.

11. I consider myself (choose one answer):

  a. Not at all homosexual

  b. Slightly homosexual

  c. Mildly homosexual

  d. Moderately homosexual

  e. Significantly homosexual

  f. Very homosexual

  g. Extremely homosexual

12. I consider myself (choose one answer):

  a. Not at all heterosexual

  b. Slightly heterosexual

  c. Mildly heterosexual

  d. Moderately heterosexual

  e. Significantly heterosexual

  f. Very heterosexual

  g. Extremely heterosexual

For additional information, see R. L. Sell, The Sell Assessment of Sexual Orientation: Background and scoring, *Archives of Sexual Behavior* 26(6) (1997): 643–58.

Gender Identity and Sex

Collecting information about assigned sex at birth (male, female) and current gender identity (e.g., man, woman, transgender, and so forth) is often referred to as the "two-step" method or approach because it uses two questions to classify respondents as transgender (discordant responses) or cisgender (concordant responses.) This approach was first developed in 1997 by the Transgender Health Advocacy Coalition, a community-based organization, for use on a survey of transgender people in Philadelphia.[73] These measures were then adapted for the Washington Transgender Needs Assessment Survey[14] and the Virginia Transgender Health Information Study.[74] A 2012 study found that the two-step approach was far more successful in identifying transgender respondents than a single, stand-alone gender identity item (which offered a transgender response option (e.g., male, female, transgender, other.)[20] Importantly, this study found that some transgender individuals identify their gender as male (or female) and not as transgender and, thus, will be overlooked if a gender identity measure is used alone.[20]

Sari Reisner and colleagues[18] evaluated a two-step approach in a predominantly white, well-educated young adult sample with the following items:

1. What sex were you assigned at birth, on your original birth certificate?
   ☐ Female
   ☐ Male

2. How do you describe yourself? (check one)
   ☐ Female
   ☐ Male
   ☐ Transgender
   ☐ Do not identify as female, male, or transgender

Cognitive testing interview participants (N=39), both cisgender (n=30) and transgender (n=9), found the items easy to understand and the response options acceptable. Quantitative analyses (n=7,833) provided evidence in support of the construct validity of the measurement approach in that recalled childhood and current gender nonconformity were each higher among those classified as transgender than cisgender. Importantly, this study validated a self-reported assigned sex-at-birth measure with mother-reported birth sex and found complete agreement.

These items, including the assigned sex-at-birth item that appeared on the 2008 US National Transgender Discrimination Experiences Survey, are recommended by the GenIUSS Group due to the availability of data on their performance. However, given that the sample was somewhat homogeneous on race-ethnicity and educational attainment, and accustomed to completing surveys as participants in a longitudinal cohort study, the authors recommend additional testing in diverse samples.

The GenIUSS Group also identified as promising a gender identity measure developed by the Center of Excellence for Transgender Health at the University of California at San Francisco: meriting testing as part of a two-step classification approach. The Center of Excellence also advises leading with a measure of current gender identity (shown below), followed by a question about sex assigned at birth. The impact of question ordering on the validity of classifications (cisgender, transgender) has yet to be studied, but is an important issue for future research.

What is your current gender identity? (Check all that apply)
   ☐ Male
   ☐ Female
   ☐ Trans male/Trans man
   ☐ Trans female/Trans woman
   ☐ Genderqueer/Gender non-conforming
   ☐ Different identity (please state): _____

Considerations for the Collection of Sexual Orientation, Gender Identity, and Sex Data Outside of Population-Based Survey Contexts

Although measuring sexual orientation, gender identity, and assigned sex at birth outside of population-based survey settings (e.g., clinical care, electronic health records) is not our primary focus, we recognize that others may look to the population-based literature for guidance. Thus, in recognition of some of the fundamental differences between population-based data collection, in which anonymous, self-reported data are the norm, and other data collection contexts, we offer a few practical suggestions:

1. Sexual orientation, current gender identity, and assigned sex at birth should be self-reported and not assumed by providers or others. Thus, when possible, sexual orientation, current gender identity, and assigned sex at birth should be collected on self-administered forms.
2. When data are to be collected by others (e.g., providers), data collectors should be trained to ask questions about sexual orientation, current gender identity, and assigned sex at birth. Training should cover the purpose of data collection and data security procedures.
3. Sexual orientation, current gender identity, and assigned sex at birth should only be collected by individuals and organizations committed to data security and privacy and that have established mechanisms to maintain security and privacy at all stages of data collection, storage, and reporting. Collecting these data as part of the electronic health record may facilitate data security and ensure privacy.

In contrast, providers should never ask clients to disclose their sexual orientation, current gender identity, or assigned sex at birth in a group setting as a means through which to obtain data. If clients receive services in a group setting, it may be advisable to have them complete an anonymous self-reported socio-demographic form (i.e., where name and date of birth are not collected). Forms should be gathered and stored in a secure place and responses aggregated and reported on group service-delivery reporting forms. If forms cannot be securely stored, then information about sexual orientation, current gender identity, and assigned sex at birth should not be collected.

1. Direct service organizations should assess their needs for provider and institutional cultural competency training and address identified gaps as the presence of sexual orientation, current gender identity, and assigned sex at birth questions in data collection forms may be perceived by clients as an indication of global LGBTQ competence.
2. Technical assistance, including staff training, protocol development, and educational material for clients, should be available to direct service organizations.
3. Good clinical practice may include collecting additional information, including the client's preferred name (which may differ from her/his/their legal name), preferred gender pronouns (he, she, other-specify:____), and sex on record with a health insurer.

References

1. Berger, P. L., and Luckmann, T. 1966. *The Social Construction of Reality: A Treatise in the Sociology of Knowledge.* New York: Anchor.

2. Delgado, R., and Stefancic, J. 2013. *Critical Race Theory: The Cutting Edge.* Third ed. Philadelphia: Temple University Press.

3. Miller, K., and Ryan, J. M. 2011. *Design, Development and Testing of the NHIS Sexual Identity Question.* Centers for Disease Control and Prevention: National Center for Health Statistics.

4. Fullilove, M. T. 1998. Comment: Abandoning "race" as a variable in public health research—An idea whose time has come. *American Journal of Public Health* 88(9): 1297–98.

5. Link, B. G., and Phelan, J. C. 2001. Conceptualizing stigma. *Annual Review of Sociology* 27: 363–85.

6. Sell, R. L. 1997. Defining and measuring sexual orientation: A review. *Archives of Sexual Behavior* 26(6): 643–58.

7. Sell, R. L., and Becker, J. B. 2001. Sexual orientation data collection and progress toward Healthy People 2010. *American Journal of Public Health* 91(6): 876–82.

8. Miller, K. 2002. *Cognitive Analysis of Sexual Identity, Attraction and Behavior Questions.* Cognitive Methods Staff Working Paper Series Number 32. Centers for Disease Control and Prevention, National Center for Health Statistics.

9. Sexual Minority Assessment Research Team. 2009. *Best Practices for Asking Questions about Sexual Orientation on Surveys.* Los Angeles: The Williams Institute (UCLA).

10. Austin, S. B., et al. 2007. Making sense of sexual orientation measures: Findings from a cognitive processing study with adolescents on health survey questions. *Journal of LGBT Health Research* 3(1): 55–65.

11. Sell, R. L. *lgbtdata.com.*

12. Kammerer, N., et al. 2001. Transgender health and social service needs in the context of HIV risk. In W. Bockting and S. Kirk, eds. *Transgender and HIV: Risks, Prevention, and Care*, 39–57. Binghamton, NY: Haworth Press.

13. McGowan, C. K. 1999. *Transgender Needs Assessment*. New York City Department of Health, HIV Prevention Planning Unit.

14. Xavier, J. M. 2000. *The Washington Transgender Needs Assessment Survey: Final report for phase two*. Washington, DC: Administration for HIV/AIDS of the District of Columbia.

15. Kenagy, G. P. 2005. Transgender health: Findings from two needs-assessment studies in Philadelphia. *Health and Social Work* 30(1): 19–26.

16. Clements-Nolle, K., et al. 2001. HIV prevalence, risk behaviors, health care use, and mental health status of transgender persons: Implications for public health intervention. *American Journal of Public Health* 91(6): 915–21.

17. Reisner, S. L., et al., 2014. Comparing in-person and online survey respondents in the U.S. National Transgender Discrimination Survey: Implications for transgender health research. *LGBT Health* 1(2): 98–106.

18. Reisner, S. L., et al., Monitoring the health of transgender and other gender minority populations: Validity of natal sex and gender identity survey items in a U.S. national cohort of young adults. *BMC Public Health* 14: 1224–1234.

19. Gordon, A. R., and Meyer, I. H. 2007. Gender nonconformity as a target of prejudice, discrimination, and violence against LGB individuals. *Journal of LGBT Health Research* 3(3): 55–71.

20. Tate, C. C., Ledbetter, J. N., and Youssef, C. P. 2013. A two-question method for assessing gender categories in the social and medical sciences. *Journal of Sex Research* 50(8): 767–76.

21. Conron, K. J., Scout, and Austin, S. B. "Everyone has a right to, like, check their box:" Findings on a measure of gender identity from a cognitive testing study with adolescents. *Journal of LGBT Health Research* 4(1): 1–9.

22. Conron, K. J. 2009. Considerations: Collecting data on transgender status and gender nonconformity. In L. Badgett and N. Goldberg, eds., *Best Practices for Asking Questions about Sexual Orientation on Surveys*, 33–37. Los Angeles: Sexual Minority Assessment Research Team, Williams Project, UCLA.

23. Wylie, S. A., et al. 2010. Socially assigned gender nonconformity: A brief measure for use in surveillance and investigation of health disparities. *Sex Roles: A Journal of Research* 63(3–4): 264–76.

24. Clark, M. A., Armstrong, G., and Bonacore, L. 2005. Measuring sexual orientation and gender expression among middle-aged and older women in a cancer screening study. *Journal of Cancer Education* 20(2): 108–12.

25. Grant, J. M., et al. 2011. *Injustice at Every Turn: A Report of the National Transgender Discrimination Survey*. Washington, DC: National Center for Transgender Equality and National Gay and Lesbian Task Force.

26. GenIUSS. 2014. *Best Practices for Asking Questions to Identify Transgender and Other Gender Minority Respondents on Population-Based Surveys*, ed. J. Heyman. Los Angeles: Williams Institute.

27. Katz, J. 1983. *Gay/Lesbian Almanac: A New Documentary in Which Is Contained, in Chronological Order, Evidence of the True and Fantastical History of Those Persons Now Called Lesbians and Gay Men*. New York: Harper & Row.

28. Ulrichs, K. H. 1994. *The Riddle of "Man-Manly" Love: The Pioneering Work on Male Homosexuality*. Buffalo, NY: Prometheus Books.

29. Prime-Stevenson, E. 1908. *The Intersexes: A History of Similisexualism as a Problem in Social Life*. Privately printed.

30. Moll, A. 1899. *Die konträre Sexualempfindung*. Berlin: Fischer's Medicin Buchhandlung.

31. Westphal K. 1869. Die kontrare Sexualempfindung: Symptom eines neuropathologischen (psychopalhischen) Zustandes. *Archiv for Psychiatrie und Nervenkrankheiten* 2: 73–108.

32. Symonds, J. A. 1889. *A Problem in Greek Ethics*. London: Privately printed.

33. Symonds, J. A. 1891. *A Problem in Modern Ethics*. London: Privately printed.

34. Krafft-Ebing, R. von 1887. *Psychopathia sexualis: Mit besonderer Berücksichtigung der conträren Sexualempfindung: Eine klinisch-forensische Studie*. Stuttgart: Ferdinand Enke

35. Carpenter E. 1894. *Homogenic Love and Its Place in a Free Society*. Manchester: Labour Press.

36. Carpenter, E. 1909. *The Intermediate Sex: A Study of Some Transitional Types of Men and Women*. 2nd ed. London: S. Sonnenschein.

37. Ellis, H. 1898. *A Note on the Bedborough Trial*. London: University Press.

38. Robinson, V. 1936. *Encyclopaedia Sexualis: A Comprehensive Encyclopaedia-Dictionary of the Sexual Sciences*. New York: Dingwall-Rock.

39. Boswell, J. 2009. *Christianity, Social Tolerance, and Homosexuality: Gay People in Western Europe from the Beginning of the Christian Era to the Fourteenth Century*. Chicago: University of Chicago Press.

40. Sell, R. L., and Petrulio, C. 1996. Sampling homosexuals, bisexuals, gays, and lesbians for public health research: A review of the literature from 1990 to 1992. *Journal of Homosexuality* 30(4): 31–47.

41. Kinsey, A. C., Pomeroy, W. B., and Martin, C. E. 1948. *Sexual Behavior in the Human Male*. New York: Ishi Press.

42. Legman, G. 1941. The language of homosexuality: An American glossary. In *Sex Variants: A Study of Homosexual Patterns*, ed. G. Henry, 1149–79. New York: Hoeber.

43. Brett, P., Wood, E., and Thomas, G. 2006. *Queering the Pitch: The New Gay and Lesbian Musicology*. New York: Routledge.

44. Signorile, M. 1993. *Queer in America*. New York: Random House.

45. Penney, J. 2014. *After Queer Theory: The Limits of Sexual Politics*. London: Pluto Press.

46. Ellis, H., and Symonds, J. A. 1998. From *Sexual Inversion* (1897). In *The Columbia Anthology of Gay Literature: Readings from Western Antiquity to the Present Day*, ed. B. R. S. Fone. New York: Columbia University Press, 1998.

47. Blumer, G. A. 1882. A case of perverted sexual instinct. *American Journal of Psychiatry* 39(1): 22–35.

48. Shaw, J. C., and Ferris, G. 1883. Perverted sexual instinct. *Journal of Nervous and Mental Disease* 10(2): 185–204.

49. Forel, A. 1908. *The Sexual Question*. London: Rebman.

50. LeVay, S. 1994. *The Sexual Brain*. Cambridge, MA: MIT Press.

51. LeVay, S. 1996. *Queer Science: The Use and Abuse of Research into Homosexuality*. Cambridge, MA: MIT Press.

52. Weinrich, J. D. 1994. Homosexuality. In *Human Sexuality: An Encyclopedia*, ed. V. Bullough and B. Bullough. New York: Garland.

53. Francoeur, R. T., and Perper, T. 1991. *A Descriptive Dictionary and Atlas of Sexology*. New York: Greenwood Press.

54. Roland, C. G. 1973. Stedman's Medical Dictionary. *Archives of Dermatology* 107(1): 130.

55. Gide, A., 1950. *Corydon*, ed. and trans. F. A. Beach and H. Gibb. New York: Farrar, Straus & Co.

56. Gonsiorek, J. C., and Weinrich, J. D. 1991. *Homosexuality: Research Implications for Public Policy*. Newbury Park, CA: Sage Publications.

57. Krieger, N. 2003. Genders, sexes, and health: What are the connections—and why does it matter? *International Journal of Epidemiology* 32(4): 652–57.

58. Conron, K. J., et al. 2014. Sex and gender in the US health surveillance system: A call to action. *American Journal of Public Health* 104(6): 970–76.

59. Barrington, D. S., et al. 2010. Racial/ethnic disparities in obesity among US-born and foreign-born adults by sex and education. *Obesity* 18(2): 422–24.

60. Ma, J., et al. 2011. Body mass index in young adulthood and premature death: Analyses of the US national health interview survey linked mortality files. *American Journal of Epidemiology* 174(8): 934–44.

61. Spence, J. T. 2011. Off with the old, on with the new. *Psychology of Women Quarterly* 35(3): 504–9.

62. US Department of Health and Human Services. 2001. *A Provider's Introduction to Substance Abuse Treatment for Lesbian, Gay, Bisexual, and Transgender Individuals*. Rockville, MD: Substance Abuse and Mental Health Services Administration

63. Feinberg, L. 1996. *Transgender Warriors: Making History from Joan of Arc to Dennis Rodman*. Boston: Beacon Press

64. Kinsey, A. C., et al. 1953. *Sexual Behavior in the Human Female*. Philadelphia, PA: Saunders.

65. Masters, W. H., and Johnson, V. E. 1979. *Homosexuality in Perspective*. Boston: Little, Brown.

66. Klein, F., B. Sepekoff, and Wolf, T. J. 1985. Sexual orientation: A multivariable dynamic process. *Journal of Homosexuality* 11(1–2): 35–49.

67. Sell, R. L., and Petrulio, C. 1996. Sampling homosexuals, bisexuals, gays, and lesbians for public health research: A review of the literature from 1990 to 1992. *Journal of Homosexuality* 30(4): 31–47.

68. Gruber, K. J., and Powers, W. A. 1982. Factor and discriminant analysis of the Bem Sex-Role Inventory. *Journal of Personality Assessment* 46(3): 284–91.

69. Bullough V. 1990. The Kinsey Scale in historical perspective. In *Homosexuality/Heterosexuality: Concepts of Sexual Orientation*, ed. D. P. McWhirter, S. A. E. Sanders, and J. M. E. Reinisch. New York: Oxford University Press.

70. Shively, M. G., and De Cecco, J. P. 1977. Components of sexual identity. *Journal of Homosexuality* 3(1): 41–48.

71. Shively, M. G., Jones, C., and De Cecco, J. P. 1984. Research on sexual orientation: Definitions and methods. *Journal of Homosexuality* 9(2–3): 127–36.

72. Sell, R. L. 1996. The Sell Assessment of Sexual Orientation: Background and scoring. *Journal of Lesbian, Gay and Bisexual Identity* 1(4): 295–310.

73. Singer, T. B., Cochran, M., and Adamec, R. 1997. *Final Report by the Transgender Health Action Coalition (THAC) to the Philadelphia Foundation Legacy Fund [for the] Needs Assessment Survey Project (a.k.a. the Delaware Valley Transgender Survey)*. Philadelphia, PA: Transgender Health Action Coalition

74. Xavier, J., Honnold, J. A., and Bradford, J. 2007. *The Health, Health-Related Needs, and Lifecourse Experiences of Transgender Virginians*. Richmond: Virginia Department of Health, Division of Disease Prevention.

FIVE

Sampling Considerations for LGBTQ Health Research

Christopher Owens, Ron Stall, and Brian Dodge

RESEARCH STUDIES on sexual and gender minority populations have used a wide range of sampling methods. *Sampling theory* posits that researchers need to define the target population, specify the sampling frame, select the sampling method and understand its limitations, determine sample size, and stratify the sample. The *sampling frame* is a set of items or elements forming the population (e.g., names, phone numbers, home addresses). *Sampling methods* are based broadly on probability and nonprobability, and *limitation* could include cost, time, generalizability, and bias. *Stratification* is a process of dividing the population into homogenous subgroups called strata; independent samples are then collected from each stratum.

Probability or Population-Based Sampling

In probability sampling, commonly known as random sampling, everyone in the sampling frame has an equal chance, or nonzero probability, of being in the sample. This randomization and equal chance allow for the sample to be representative, allow results to be generalized to the population sampled, and facilitate less bias. However, probability sampling has limitations: it is costly, and LGBT-identified individuals represent only an estimated 1%–4% of the US population.

One option to solve these limitations is to use subsets of national or state cross-sectional questionnaires that include questions about sexual orientation and gender identity, behavior, and attraction. Since certain national- and state-level surveys use probability sampling, data disaggregated by LGBTQ respondents can be generalized. Several federal and state surveys use questions related to sexual orientation and gender identity, behavior, or attraction: the Behavioral Risk Factor Surveillance System, the California Health Interview Survey, the National Epidemiological Survey on Alcohol and Related Conditions, the National Health and Nutrition Examination Study, the National Health and Social Life Survey, the National Health Interview Survey, the National Household Survey on Drug Abuse, the National Survey of Family Growth, the National Survey of Sexual Health and Behavior, and the Youth Risk Behavior Surveillance System. Although these studies use questions related to sexual orientation and gender identity, behavior, and attraction, nationally representative studies include few respondents who identify as LGBTQ, and they cannot address variability between and among LGBTQ populations (e.g., racial/ethnical groups). State-level cross-sectional surveys may have more LGBTQ respondents. Cochran and Mays (2009) analyzed data from the 2003 California Health Interview Survey and the 2004–2005 California Quality of Life Survey regarding psychiatric morbidity among LGB Californians. The California Health Interview Survey uses random-digit dialing and is a structured computer-assisted telephone interview. Cochran and Mays analyzed 652 sexual minorities ages 18–72 from the sample of 2,272 Californians, measuring psychiatric morbidity from the Composite International Diagnostic Interviews Short Form and the Kessler Psychological Distress Scale. LGBTQ health researchers can also gather nationally representative data by collaborating with research panel organizations or by using their collected data.

Online probability research panels are another probability data collection method for nationally representative, population-based sampling. One advantage of using research panels is that their data are nationally representative and that this sample is collected for you (or already collected for you if you are using a previously collected research panel). A disadvantage, as with the national- and state-level surveys, is that the sample may include few respondents who identify as LGBTQ. Since 2010, researchers at Indiana University have used GfK/Knowledge Networks to conduct the annual National Survey of Sexual Health and Behavior (NSSHB), including a focus on the general population of gay, lesbian, bisexual, and other sexual minority groups in the United States (Reece et al. 2010, Dodge et al. 2016). The NSSHB is a population-based cross-sectional survey measuring recent and lifetime prevalence of sexual behaviors among adolescents and adults in the United States. Knowledge Networks used the US Postal Service's Delivery Sequence File and the Current Population Survey to obtain a sampling frame that covers approximately 98% of all US households. Once panels were established, Knowledge Networks invited those in the panels to participate in the NSSHB. Data were collected online, and panel members were provided internet access if needed. This resulted in a nationally representative probability sample of 5,865 men and women ages 14–94.

Nonprobability Sampling

In *nonprobability sampling*, commonly called convenience sampling, the probability of a person selected to participate is unknown and requires no randomization among the sample. This lack of randomization produces participant bias and nongeneralizable results. However, nonprobability studies have provided insights into health among LGBTQ populations (Institute of Medicine 2011), and nonprobability methods are quicker and less costly than probability methods. Nonprobability sampling is often used if a researcher does not have resources to conduct a probability sample study (due, for example, to constraints of time, finances, or personnel) or has a defined and small study population. Commonly used nonprobability sampling methods include convenience, community or neighborhood, venue-based, and snowball (or peer-referral) sampling. Each of these nonprobability techniques requires different processes. Meyer and Wilson (2009) observed that "for most nonprobability sampling procedures, 'convenience' is a misnomer; non-probability sampling requires very careful consideration, design, and execution" (p. 26).

LGBTQ health researchers can use *neighborhood sampling* to identify and target geographical areas that have a greater proportion of LGBTQ-identified individuals. LGBTQ health researchers use representative survey results to facilitate a greater sample of LGBTQ respondents through neighborhood sampling. For example, Bye et al. (2005) used data from the 2000 Census to identify areas with high proportions of LGBTQ-identified individuals. They then used a disproportionate stratified and random-digit dialing (RDD) sampling design to collect data on tobacco use and attitudes among LGBTQ-identified people living in six stratum areas. Catania et al.'s Urban Men's Health Study (2001), also using RDD, targeted MSM who lived in specific Chicago, Los Angeles, New York, and San Francisco neighborhoods. Meyer and Wilson (2009, p. 25) noted the limitations of neighborhood sampling: "When sampling LGB neighborhoods, researchers explicitly or implicitly assume that individuals in their sample are similar to LGBs not residing in such neighborhoods, but this is not a safe assumption. Compared with nonresidents, LGBTs residing in LGB neighborhoods probably are . . . of higher income and social class. . . . Although the greatest benefit of probability sampling is in generalization, the modification to targeted neighborhood compromises this main benefit."

Respondent-Driven Sampling

Designed for sampling hidden populations, *respondent-driven sampling* (RDS) combines snowball sampling with a mathematical model. Like snowball sampling, RDS is a chain-referral method in which existing study subjects recruit future subjects in their social networks who meet eligibility criteria. Unlike snowball sampling, RDS uses a two-tiered incentive system and can make unbiased population estimates (like probability sampling). All participants receive compensation for participating, but participants can receive additional incentives by recruiting peers to participate in the study. Original respondents (called seeds) are given coupons to recruit peers who meet specific eligibility criteria. A referral (called a recruiter) presents their coupon, and the seed receives an additional incentive. The recruiter also receives the dual-incentive plan and can recruit people in their social networks. One disadvantage of RDS is that it assumes that original respondents recruit their referrals at random. Two solutions are to ensure that the first-wave respondents are diverse and to sensitize recruitment (such as asking the recruiter how they know the seed).

Venue-Based and Time-Space Sampling

Venue-based sampling refers to sampling venues where researchers believe LGBTQ people congregate or where LGBTQ people can be identified. For example, researchers can conduct venue-based sampling at LBGT bars/clubs, social groups, and Pride events. Meyer and Wilson (2009, p. 26) noted one weakness of this sampling method: "This approach can only reach LGB persons who partake in the LGB community, overlooking individuals who are not identified as LGB. . . . Individuals who do not partake in the LGB community are different from those who do." This means that participant bias is prominent in venue-based sampling. One alternative to venue-based sampling is to conduct *time-space sampling* (TSS, also known as venue-based, time-space sampling). TSS could assert randomization over venues and times of data collection, thus increasing the generalization of findings. First, researchers identify and select venues in which the target population congregates, often through ethnographic assessments, key informant interviews, or focus groups. These informants and researchers create a comprehensive set of sites where LGBTQ people are situated—unlike venue-based sampling, where researchers speculate as to where LGBTQ people are situated. Second, researchers attend sites at random times to record demographic patterns. These data create the time-space unit sampling frame. The time-space unit is a day and time when the target population visits that venue. Third, researchers randomly select time-space units to recruit participants. Time-space sampling has several advantages over other sampling methods: it encourages community participation; it decreases bias (since it draws on probability-based methods of randomization); and it increases the generalizability of findings.

Nonprobability Web-Based Sampling

In *web-based sampling*, also called online or internet-based sampling, LGBTQ researchers recruit participants and distribute a cross-sectional questionnaire on the internet, most often through websites. Although web-based sampling is relatively easy and inexpensive to administer, it runs the risk of participant bias (Grov et al. 2014) since the population of interest may not be online during the survey distribution timeframe or might even not have internet access. Research has shown there is a digital divide in internet usage in the United States: Americans who use the internet are often younger, have higher socioeconomic status, and are whiter than Americans without internet access. To decrease bias, LGBTQ health researchers can incorporate other sampling methodologies such as probability and venue-based sampling. They can also use previous online research panels, such as Knowledge Networks listed above, to collect a more rigorous probability-based sample. Of course, like nationally representative cross-sectional surveys, these previously collected research panels may include few respondents who identify as LGBTQ and thus fail to reflect diversity within the LGBTQ population. LGBTQ health researchers can conduct a cyber-ethnography (also called virtual ethnography or online ethnography) of potential websites as recruitment venues (Carballo-Dieguez et al. 2006). LGBTQ health researchers use cyber-ethnography to describe the website and online community characteristics, and then later infer whether that website will be used as a recruitment venue based on the population and measures of interests.

The decision on which sampling method to choose depends on the research question, study constraints, and sampling theory components. For example, if a researcher is interested in evaluating risks for HIV/AIDS among MSM, then a venue-based sampling among public sex environments, online geosocial networking apps, and bathhouses might be more appropriate than other sampling methods. If a researcher is interested in evaluating tobacco norms among transgender youth, then RDS might be more useful than other sampling methods. Study resources and constraints will determine sampling method. Researchers commonly use nonprobability sampling due to study constraints such as lack of access to probability research panels, time, and money. If a researcher does not have sufficient funds for incentives, then a nonprobability online sampling method may be cheaper than RDS. The sampling frame will define the population of interest, and access to this population will inform the choice of sampling method. LGBTQ health researchers must appraise the strengths and weaknesses of sampling methods under consideration; because each method has strengths and weaknesses, no standard method applies to LGBTQ health research.

Which Sampling Method Is Best for My Study?

One of the most challenging decisions in designing research with LGBTQ populations is selecting a sampling method. This decision is generally regarded as one of the central qualities for judging the scientific rigor of a study, with population-based sampling methods typically regarded as being the most rigorous. The choice of sampling method thus becomes particularly charged given that adhering to protocols designed for sampling from the general population can become quite difficult when applied to relatively rare, hidden, or disadvantaged populations, as is often the case with sexual minorities.

Commentaries on sampling methods are often framed in terms of a hierarchy in regards to methodological rigor: methods that use convenience samples are often discussed as if they are intrinsically less rigorous than those that use probability methods to recruit subjects. We would argue that sampling frames that use probability methods certainly have strong methodological advantages, but that these are not the only factors that should be considered in terms of choosing a sampling method for LGBTQ populations. Further, it is possible to make a strong argument that privileging randomized sampling techniques ignores the many costs of using these methods, and an over-reliance on these methods may actually impede moving the field of LGBTQ health forward. Regardless of study design, there is always a possibility of bias, fallacy, and lack of casual association.

(continued)

We would also argue for a broader definition of methodological rigor that is *not* achieved through consideration of one aspect of study design alone (as might be the case in terms of sampling methods), but rather is achieved when the investigator successfully achieves a balance between a number of methodological concerns. These concerns include the ability to expand theoretical understandings of LGBTQ health, cost, feasibility; the ability to focus on areas specific to sexual minorities; and the ability to recruit large numbers of subjects and so conduct highly powered analyses, among other criteria.

We provide below a simplified summary—and perhaps an oversimplification—of how these criteria typically perform across a range of sampling methods. For example, in an area of research that is only now receiving scientific attention but for which we know there is very likely to be a health disparity, a convenience sampling approach may be the most rigorous choice. This is because this study could be put into the field while allowing for the ability to include theoretically innovative measures and to include measures that tap the lived experiences of LGBTQ populations, all with a high degree of feasibility, the possibility of including large numbers of subjects, and at relatively low cost. On the other hand, if multiple convenience sample analyses have already been published, and there is still some doubt as to whether a specific disparity exists within a specific LGBTQ population, a general population sampling strategy would likely make the greatest contribution to the field. This is because by using a general population sampling strategy, we can move toward settling the question of whether a disparity exists and proceed to the issue of understanding the factors that give rise to this disparity.

Note that this general schema assumes that there is a conversation between studies, and that given the general level of research and data to explain a particular health disparity, different sampling strategies can assume greater or lesser rigor as the field of study evolves. Thus, the rigor of a study should be judged not only in terms of the operational aspects of completing the study, but also how it contributes to our understandings of how to best address particular disparities and so move the larger field forward.

So how does one pick a sampling strategy? In the end, we would argue that the primary criterion is not one of supposed rigor according to a supposed methodological purity, but rather an expanded definition of rigor that is based on a balance of blending a set of important theoretical and public health–impact considerations that together best move the field forward.

Table 5.1 Considerations in Choosing a Sampling Strategy for a Descriptive Study of LGBTQ Populations

Sampling Strategy	Theoretical Creativity	Perceived Rigor	Cost	Feasibility	Measures Specific to Sexual Minorities	Large N
Convenience-Venue	High	Low	Low	High	High	Possible
Convenience-Internet	High	Generally low	Relatively low	Relatively high	High	Possible
Time-Space	High	Can be high	Moderately expensive	Depends on circumstances	High	Possible
Respondent-Driven Sampling	Can be high	Can be high	Moderately expensive	Depends on circumstances	High	Can be achieved
Random-Digit Dial	Can be high	Can be high	Can be expensive	Becoming difficult	Can be high	Can be achieved
Neighborhood Population	Can be high	Can be high	Likely to be expensive	Difficult to field	Can be high	Difficult to achieve
National Population	Difficult to achieve due to cost	Very high	Very expensive	Difficult to field	Generally low	Very difficult to achieve

So, which is the best sampling method? In the end, it depends on your research question, the scientific context in which your question was formed, and the resources available to address your question. If you meet the balance of theoretical innovation, public health impact, and operational rigor in defining the sampling method that you will use, you are likely to be able to move the field forward in important ways. We recommend being familiar with the strengths and limitations of sampling methods you are considering, and that you talk with advisors, peers, and others to gain input on which sampling method is best to address your criteria.

References

Bostwick, W. B., Hughes, T. L., and Everett, B. 2015. Health behavior, status, and outcomes among a community-based sample of lesbian and bisexual women. *LGBT Health* 2(2): 121–26.

Bradford, J., Reisner, S. L., Honnold, J. A., and Xavier, J. 2013. Experiences of transgender-related discrimination and implications for health: Results from the Virginia Transgender Health Initiative Study. *American Journal of Public Health* 103(10): 1820–29.

Bryant, L., Damarin, A. K., and Marshall, Z. 2014. Tobacco control recommendations identified by LGBT Atlantans in a Community-Based Participatory Research Project. *Progress in Community Health Partnerships: Research, Education, and Action* 8(3): 269–79.

Burkhalter, J. E., Hay, J. L., Coups, E., Warren, B., Li, Y., and Ostroff, J. S. 2011. Perceived risk for cancer in an urban sexual minority. *Journal of Behavioral Medicine* 34(3): 157–69.

Bye, L., Gruskin, E., Greenwood, G., Albright, V., and Krotki, K. 2005. *California Lesbians, Gays, Bisexuals, and Transgender Tobacco Use Survey—2004*. Sacramento, CA: California Department of Health Services.

Carballo-Diéguez, A., Dowsett, G. W., Ventuneac, A., Remien, R. H., Balan, I., Dolezal, C., Luciano, O., and Lin P. 2006. Cybercartography of popular internet sites used by New York City men who have sex with men interested in bareback sex. *AIDS Education and Prevention* 18(6): 475–89.

Catania, J., Osmond, D., Stall, R. D., Pollack, L., Paul, J. P., Blower, S. . . . Coates, T. J. 2001. The continuing HIV epidemic among men who have sex with men. *American Journal of Public Health* 91(6): 907–14.

Choi, K. H., Han, C. S., Hudes, E. S., and Kegeles, S. 2002. Unprotected sex and associated risk factors among young Asian and Pacific Islander men who have sex with men. *AIDS Education and Prevention* 14(6): 472–81.

Clements-Nolle, K., Marx, R., and Katz, M. 2006. Attempted suicide among transgender persons. *Journal of Homosexuality* 51(3): 53–69.

Clements-Nolle, K., Marx, R., Guzman, R., and Katz, M. 2001. HIV prevalence, risk behaviors, health care use, and mental health status of transgender persons: Implications for public health intervention. *American Journal of Public Health* 91(6): 915–21.

Cochran, S. D., and Mays, V. M. 2009. Burden of psychiatric morbidity among lesbian, gay, and bisexual individuals in the California Quality of Life Survey. *Journal of Abnormal Psychology* 118(3): 647–58.

De Haan, G., Santos, G. M., Arayasirikul, S., and Raymond, H. F. 2015. Non-prescribed hormone use and barriers to care for transgender women in San Francisco. *LGBT Health* 2(4), 313–23.

Dodge, B., Herbenick, D., Fu., T., Schick, V., Reece, M., Sanders, S. A., and Fortenberry, J. D. 2016. Sexual behaviors of U.S. men by self-identified sexual orientation: Results from the 2012 National Survey of Sexual Behavior. *Journal of Sexual Medicine* 13(4): 637–49.

Eaton, L. A., Matthews, D. D., Driffin, D. D., Bukowski, L., Wilson, P. A., Stall, R. D., and Team, T. P. 2017. A multi-US city assessment of awareness and uptake of pre-exposure prophylaxis (PrEP) for HIV prevention among black men and transgender women have sex with men. *Prevention Science* 18(5): 505–16

Fallin, A., Neilands, T. B., Jordan, J. W., and Ling, P. M. 2014. Secondhand smoke exposure among young adult sexual minority bar and nightclub patrons. *American Journal of Public Health* 104(2): 148–53.

Gallagher, K. M., Sullivan, P. S., Lansky, A., and Onorato, I. M. 2007. Behavioral surveillance among people at risk for HIV infection in the U.S.: The National HIV Behavioral Surveillance System. *Public Health Report* 122(1): 32–38.

Grant, J. M., Mottet, L. A., Tanis, J., Herman, J. L., Harrison, J., and Keisling, M. 2010. *National Transgender Discrimination Survey Report on Health and Health Care.* Washington, DC: National Center for Transgender Equality and the National Gay and Lesbian Task Force (http://www.thetaskforce.org).

Grov, C., Breslow, A. S., Newcomb, M. E., Rosenberger, J. G., and Bauermeister, J. A. 2014. Gay and Bisexual men's use of the Internet: Research from the 1990s through 2013. *Journal of Sex Research* 51(4): 390–409.

Herek, G. M., Gillis, J. R., and Cogan, J. C. 1999. Psychological sequelae of hate-crime victimization among lesbian, gay, and bisexual adults. *Journal of Counseling and Clinical Psychology* 67(6): 945–51.

Institute of Medicine. 2011. Conducting research on the health status of LBGT populations. Chapter 3 in *The Health of Lesbian, Gay, Bisexual and Transgender Population: Building a Foundation for Better Understanding,* 89–140. Washington, DC: National Academies Press.

Lee, J. G., Goldstein, A. O., Ranney, L. M., Crist, J., and McCullough, A. 2011. High tobacco use among lesbian, gay, and bisexual populations in West Virginian bars and community festivals. *International Journal of Environmental Research and Public Health* 8(7): 2758–69.

Logie, C. H., Lacombe-Duncan, A., Weaver, J., Navia, D., and Este, D. 2015. A pilot study of a group-based HIV and STI prevention intervention for lesbian, bisexual, queer, and other women who have sex with women in Canada. *AIDS Patient Care* 29(6): 321–28.

Martin, J. L., and Dean, L. 1990. Developing a community sample of gay men for an epidemiologic study of AIDS. *American Behavioral Scientist* 33(5): 546–61.

Meyer, I. H., and Wilson, P. A. 2009. Sampling lesbian, gay, and bisexual populations. *Journal of Counseling Psychology* 56(1): 23–31.

Meyer, I. H., Dietrich, J., and Schwartz, S. 2008. Lifetime prevalence of mental disorders and suicide attempts in diverse lesbian, gay, and bisexual populations. *American Journal of Public Health* 98(6): 1004–6.

Meyer, I. H., Schwartz, S., and Frost, D. M. 2008. Social patterning of stress and coping: Does disadvantaged social statuses confer more stress and fewer coping resources? *Social Science & Medicine* 67(3): 368–79.

Meyer, I. H., Teylan, M., and Schwartz, S. 2015. The role of help-seeking in preventing suicide attempts among lesbians, gay men, and bisexuals. *Suicide and Life-Threatening Behavior* 45(1): 25–36.

Mills, T. C., Stall, R., Pollack, L., Paul, J. P., Binson, D., Canchola, J., and Catania, J. A. 2001. Health-related characteristics of men who have sex with men: A comparison of those living in "gay ghettos" with those living elsewhere. *American Journal of Public Health,* 91(6): 980–83.

Mimiaga, M. J., Case, P., Johnson, C. V., Safren, S. A., and Mayer, K. H. 2009. Pre-exposure antiretroviral prophylaxis (PrEP) attitudes in high risk Boston area

MSM: Limited knowledge and experience, but potential for increased utilization after education. *Journal of Acquired Immune Deficiency Syndromes* 50(1): 77–83.

Mimiaga, M. J., Reisner, S. L., Cranston, K., Isenberg, D., Bright, D., Daffin G., . . . Mayer, K. H. (2009). Sexual mixing patterns and partner characteristics of Black MSM in Massachusetts at increased risk for HIV infection and transmission. *Journal of Urban Health* 86(4): 602–23.

Morgan, E., Skaathum, B., Michaels, S., Young, L., Khanna, A., Friedman, S. R., . . . Team, T. U. 2016. Marijuana use as a sex-drug is associated with HIV risk among Black MSM and their networks. *AIDS and Behavior* 20(3): 600–607.

Morris, J. F., and Rothblum, E. D. 1999. Who fills out a "lesbian" questionnaire? The interrelationship of sexual orientation, years "out," disclosure of sexual orientation, sexual experience with women, and participation in the lesbian community. *Psychology of Women Quarterly* 23(3): 537–57.

Mustanski, B., and Liu, R. T. 2013. A longitudinal study of predictors of suicide attempts among lesbian, gay, bisexual, and transgender youth. *Archives of Sexual Behavior* 42(3): 437–48.

Mustanski, B., Ryan, D. T., and Garofalo, R. 2014. Associations of sexually transmitted infections with condom problems among young men who have sex with men. *Sexually Transmitted Diseases* 41(7): 427–32.

Operario, D., and Nemoto, T. 2005. Sexual risk behavior and substance use among a sample of Asian Pacific Islander transgendered women. *AIDS Education and Prevention* 17(5): 430–43.

Patel, V. V., Masyukova, M., Sutton, D., and Horvath, K. J. 2016. Social media use and HIV-related risk behaviors in young Black and Latino gay and bi men and transgender individuals in New York City: Implications for online interventions. *Journal of Urban Health* 93(2): 388–99.

Reece, M., Herbenick, D., Schick, V., Sanders, S. A., Dodge, B., and Fortenberry, J. D. 2010. Background and considerations on the National Survey of Sexual Health and Behavior (NSSHB) from investigators. *Journal of Sexual Medicine* 7(5): 243–45.

Reisner, S. L., Mimiaga, M. J., Bland, S., Skeer, M., Cranston, K., Isenberg, D., . . . Mayer, K. H. 2010. Problematic alcohol use and HIV risk among Black men who have sex with men in Massachusetts. *AIDS Care* 22(5): 577–87.

Reisner, S. L., Mimiaga, M. J., Johnson, C. V., Bland, S., Case, P., Safren, S. A., and Mayer, K. H. 2010. What makes a respondent-driven sampling "seed" productive? Example of finding at-risk Massachusetts men who have sex with men. *Journal of Urban Health* 87(3): 467–479.

Reisner, S. L., Mimiaga, M. J., Skeer, M., Bright, D., Cranston, K., Isenberg, D., . . . Mayer, K. H. 2009. Clinically significant depressive symptoms as a risk factor for HIV infection among Black MSM in Massachusetts. *AIDS and Behavior* 13(4): 798–810.

Reisner, S., Mimiaga, M., Bland, S. E., Driscoll, M. A., Cranston, K., and Mayer, K. H. 2012. Pathways to embodiment of HIV risk: Black men who have sex with transgender partners, Boston, Massachusetts. *AIDS Education and Prevention* 24(1): 15–26.

Remafedi, G., Jurek, A. M., and Oakes, M. 2008. Sexual identity and tobacco use in a venue-based sample of adolescents and young adults. *American Journal of Preventative Medicine* 35(6): 463–70.

Robinson, B. E., Galbraith, J. S., Romie, R. E., Zhang, Q., and Herbst, J. H. 2013. Differences between HIV-positive and HIV-negative African American men who have sex with men in two major U.S. metropolitan areas. *Archives of Sexual Behavior* 42(2): 267–78.

Robinson, W. T., Brown, M. C., and Moody-Thomas, S. 2014. Smoking and experiences with tobacco cessation among men who have sex with men: New Orleans, 2011. *AIDS and Behavior* 8(3): 324–32.

Rooser, B. R., Miner, M. H., Bockting, W. O., Ross, M. W., Konstan, J. K., Gurak, L., . . . Coleman, E. 2009. HIV risk and the internet: Results of the Men's INTernet Sex (MINTS) Study. *AIDS and Behavior* 13(4): 746–56.

Ross, M. W., Berg, R. C., Schmidt, A. J., Hospers, H. J., Breveglieri, M., Furegato, M., . . . Network, T. E. 2013. Internalised homonegativity predicts HIV-associated risk behavior in European men who have sex with men in a 38-country cross-sectional study: Some public health implications of homophobia. *BMJ Open* 3(2): e001928.

Rothblum, E. D., and Factor, R. 2001. Lesbians and their sisters as control group: Demographic and mental health factors. *Psychological Sciences* 12(1): 63–69.

Santos, G. M., Rapues, J., Wilson, E. C., Macias, O., Packer, T., Colfax, G., and Raymond, H. F. 2014. Alcohol and substance use among transgender women in San Francisco: Prevalence and association with human immunodeficiency virus infection. *Drug and Alcohol Review* 33(3): 287–95.

Sapsirisavat, V., Phanuphak, N., Keadpudsa, S., Egan J. E., Pussadee, K., Klay-tong P., . . . Team, T. F. 2016. Psychological and behavioral characteristics of high-risk men who have sex with men (MSM) of unknown HIV positive serostatus in Bangkok, Thailand. *AIDS and Behavior* 20(3): 386–97.

Schneider, J., Michaels, S., and Bouris, A. 2012. Family network proportion and HIV risk among Black men who have sex with men. *Journal of Acquired Immune Deficiency Syndromes* 61(5): 627–35.

Shilo, G. S., and Mor, Z. 2014. The impact of minority stressors on the mental and physical health of lesbian, gay, and bisexual youth and young adults. *Health & Social Work* 39(3): 161–71.

Stephenson, R., and Finneran, C. 2016. Minority stress and intimate partner violence among gay and bisexual men in Atlanta. *American Journal of Men's Health* 11(4): 952–61

Stueve, A., O'Donnell, L. N., Duran, R., San Doval, A., and Blome, J. 2001. Time-space sampling in minority communities: Results with young Latino men who have sex with men. *American Journal of Public Health* 91(6): 922–26.

Thompson, H. M., Reisner, S. K., VanKim, N., and Raymond, H. F. 2015. Quality-of-life measurement: Assessing the WHOQOL-BREF scale in a sample of high-HIV-risk transgender women in San Francisco, California. *International Journal of Transgenderism* 16(1): 36–48.

Wang, J., Häusermann, M., Vounatsou, P., Aggelton, P., and Weiss, M. G. 2007. Health status, behavior, and care utilization in the Geneva Gay Men's Health Survey. *Preventive Medicine* 44(1): 70–75.

White, J. M., Mimiaga, M. J., Reisner, S. L., and Mayer, K. H. 2013. HIV sexual risk behavior among Black men who meet other men on the internet for sex. *Journal of Urban Health* 90(3): 464–81.

Xavier, J. M., Bobbin, M., Singer, B., and Budd, E. 2005. A needs assessment of Transgendered people of color living in Washington, D.C. *International Journal of Transgenderism*, 8(2/3): 3–47.

SIX

Theory as a Practical Tool in Research and Intervention

Ilan H. Meyer, with the Generations Study Investigators

When I used to teach a Health Psychology class to public health students, before getting to the theories section, I had to convince students to find theories relevant. I had to convince them to go against their intuition, which told them that what is meaningful is what we do in public health—intervene and have an impact on real-world problems—not contemplating theoretical propositions. In the first session of the section, I used to quote Kurt Lewin (1952) who said, "there is nothing as practical as a good theory" (p. 169). This quote hides a double-edged admonition to researchers: "theorists should strive to create theories that can be used to solve social or practical problems, and practitioners and researchers . . . should make use of available scientific theory."

Vansteenkiste and Sheldon 2006, 63

ONE IMPORTANT way theories are useful is that they tell us where to look for causal relationships. Theory can direct us to intervene where our intervention may have the most impact because theory helps us identify the causes of a problem we want to address. Theories are also useful in that, usually, they take a broader view of the issues than what may be tackled in any one research or intervention project. For example, theory can help identify the fundamental cause of a problem at hand and assess whether that is a feasible point of intervention (Link and Phelan 1995; Meyer and Frost 2013).

The theory of minority stress, which I discuss here, describes various causes at various levels (structural and interpersonal). But any risk-factors or intervention researcher may choose to focus on a subset of these causes or levels. Thus, in any particular research or intervention project, a theory can not only help researchers identify what to focus on; it also reminds us of other potential causes that we are *not* focusing on. As we assess the model we are using, we can thus better estimate which effects to expect because we can also estimate which effects will continue to impact the outcomes unaffected by our intervention. In research, this is important because it will help us better articulate (or *specify*) our causal model; in interventions, this is important because we can better estimate the total impact of the intervention on the target outcome.

The Origins of Minority Stress Theory

I started to develop the basic principles of minority stress as a graduate student working on my dissertation. Theoretical thinking determined the direction that my work took before I could see the full picture or what that direction would be. In the late 1980s, I started with the observation that homophobia would have a negative psychological impact on LGB people. This was not a big stretch of imagination: LGB affirmative psychology had described the toll of homophobia on LGB people and the importance of coming out as a way of releasing one's self from internalized negative perception of one's homosexuality. Indeed, clinical writers at the time had identified internalized homophobia as one of the most important issues to address in therapy with LGB clients (Maylon 1982). But it is important to remember that at the time I was developing my ideas about the negative impact of stress related to homophobia, there was no focus on health disparities with which we are so familiar today in US public health. Although minority stress has become the most commonly used explanation of health disparities between sexual minorities and heterosexuals, this focus did not emerge until about 2000. Indeed, most psychological literature on LGB people prior to the late 1990s had asserted that LGB people (research did not often explicitly discuss bisexuals) were as mentally, and certainly physically, healthy as straight people.

This claim—that there were no disparities in mental health between LGB people and heterosexuals—was, in part, a heritage of the historical debates about the status of homosexuality as a mental disorder (Bayer 1981). In the early 1970s, psychiatrists and psychologists debated whether homosexuality should remain classified as a mental disorder in the *Diagnostic and Statistical Manual of Mental Disorders (DSM)*, as it had been for decades before. The debate focused in part on whether LGB people had a higher prevalence of mental disorders (e.g., major depression disorder) than straight people. The rationale was that if LGB people have higher prevalence of mental disorders than heterosexuals, that means that homosexuality itself is a disorder and therefore should remain thus classified. It is important to note that this is flawed logic: classification of a disorder does not depend on whether people diagnosed with the purported disorder have a high prevalence of *other* mental disorders. That is, if a group has a high prevalence of a mental disorder, as is the case for women and major depression disorder, that would not make being a member of the group—that is, being a woman—itself a disorder. In the same way, whether LGB people have a high prevalence of mental disorders does not inform whether homosexuality itself should be classified as a disorder. The question of what justifies a categorization as a disorder is beyond the scope of this chapter, but clearly having a high prevalence of other disorders is not it.

One thing to note is that, during the 1970s, researchers on both sides of the debate—trying to prove that LGB people had or did not have high prevalence of disorders—relied on what we would now consider unsophisticated methods. For example, they used nonprobability samples, including clinical and prison populations, which cannot be used to estimate population prevalence without bias, and they had poor diagnostic tests. This was in part because psychiatric epidemiology was still a field in its infancy—the first large-scale psychiatric epidemiological study in the United States relying on probability samples and standardized measures started only in the 1980s (Robins and Regier, 1991).

But even though this rationale had already been debunked at the time as nonsensical (Marmor 1980), this was an important rhetoric during the debate on the status of homosexuality as a disorder. Therefore, by the 1980s, LGB-affirmative psychologists and psychiatrists repeated the assertion that has become associated with a LGB-affirmative perspective: that LGB people do *not* have a higher prevalence of mental disorders, such as depression and anxiety, compared with heterosexuals.

As I was developing ideas on minority stress, I realized that if minority stress is correct, and if stress causes disorders, then LGB people would have a higher prevalence of disorders than heterosexuals. So either the minority stress theory is wrong or the evidence on the mental health of LGB people is wrong. I had to decide whether I should be loyal to the theory or to the received LGB-affirmative view. At the time, this caused an ethical dilemma: Do I pursue what I think is correct based on theories of prejudice and stigma, or should I endorse the supposedly LGB-affirmative perspective and abandon my work as incompatible with the research evidence?

Theory won. I was convinced by the work of many traditions in psychology, sociology, and public health: Minority stress was informed by theories of prejudice (Allport 1954), stigma (Goffman 1963), and many stress researchers (Dohrenwend 1998; Pearlin 1982; Holmes and Rahe 1967; Lazarus and Folkman 1984). Also importantly, I was not convinced that the LGB-affirmative notion—that there were no differences in prevalence of disorders between LGB and straight people—was the only LGB-affirmative stance. Indeed, I believed that minority stress was an LGB-affirmative theory in that it pointed to events and conditions in the world that caused harm to LGB people. The implication of minority stress is in the promise that social and legal changes that would lead to alleviating stressors related to prejudice and stigma would, in turn, lead to improved conditions, and improved health, for LGB people.

That was the context of the first paper on minority stress (Meyer 1995); since then, the discourse started to shift. In the 2000s, research evidence had begun to emerge that suggested that LGB people were indeed suffering from an excess of mental disorders compared with heterosexuals. First, in 1999, two articles were published in the journal *Archives of General Psychiatry* (Herrell et al. 1999; Fergusson, Horwood, and Beautrais 1999; because of the novelty of the findings, they were accompanied by three editorials), and later, a study from the Netherlands was published in the same journal (Sandfort, de Graaf, Bijl, and Schnabel 2001). Several articles using US national probability samples followed (Cochran and Mays 2000a; Cochran and Mays 2000b; Cochran 2001; Mays and Cochran 2001). Together, these studies showed clearly that LGB people had a higher prevalence of depression, anxiety, substance-use disorders, and suicide attempts compared with heterosexuals. At about the same time, the US Public Health Service began to focus on the problem of health disparities, which became a cornerstone of Healthy People 2010, published in 2000, and described reducing health disparities as a main national goal (US Department of Health and Human Services 2000). Together, these developments led to greater acceptance of minority stress as a framework for understanding the health of LGB people.

In 2010, Healthy People 2020 recognized disparities by gender identity in addition to sexual orientation. More recently, efforts to incorporate transgender health issues into a minority stress framework have developed as well (Hendricks and Testa 2012; Testa, Habarth, Peta, Balsam, and Bockting 2015; Bockting, Miner, Swinburne Romine, Hamilton, and Coleman 2013; Bockting et al. 2016). The theory and even the specific processes described by minority stress are relevant to both sexual and gender minorities, but there are some important distinctions. Most obviously, transgender individuals have to cope with stressors related to gender affirmation that LGB people generally do not (Sevelius 2013). It would be a mistake, however, to assume that gender, and especially gender-conformity, is irrelevant to understanding minority stress in LGB people. Indeed, same-sex sexuality is often seen as a transgression of gender roles. Prejudice and stigma related to gender nonconformity can be a major cause of stress for LGB people, including violence perpetrated against them (Gordon and Meyer 2007).

Basic Concepts in Minority Stress

I and others have described minority stress in several papers (Hendricks and Testa 2012; Meyer 1995; Meyer 2003; Meyer and Frost 2013;

Meyer 2015; Schwartz and Meyer 2010). Minority stress is a theory of causation; it states that because of prejudice and stigma, LGBTQ people are exposed to more stress than cisgender heterosexual people (everything else, like race/ethnicity and class, being equal). The theory states that prejudice and stigma directed at LGBTQ people lead to experiences of stress of various types (e.g., large-magnitude life events, everyday discrimination, chronic stressors). This stress, because it originates in prejudice and stigma specifically related to sexual and gender minority status, is unique and therefore comes in excess to the stress that all people experience. In turn, that excess stress exposure is a risk factor that leads to excess burden of disorders, including mental and physical, that are caused by stress. Because minority stress describes the cause of disorders, and because it is describing excess burden, it explains disparities in health outcomes between LGBTQ and cisgender heterosexual people.

Thus, it is important to understand that minority stress describes *excess* stress (not simply *different* stress) compared with that of cisgender heterosexual people. This is a basic epidemiological principle that explains why, for example, people who smoke (i.e., who have a higher exposure to risk) would have a higher prevalence of lung cancer than people who do not smoke. This characteristic of the minority stress model makes it a theory explaining health disparities. If minority stress only described a type of stress that is *different*, but not *additive,* to the stress that all people experience, it would not explain disparities in health.

I have often described minority stress as being *unique* stress, but the term *unique* can be confusing. Minority stress is unique not because the stressful experiences are unique but because the *source* of the stressors—sexual prejudice and stigma—are unique to sexual and gender minorities. For example, losing a job is a stressful event that is not unique to LGBTQ people—all people are at risk of experiencing it. But as a minority stressor it is unique when the loss of a job occurs due to discrimination on the basis of sexual or gender identity status. That is, people could be fired from a job for many reasons (shrinking of the job market, unsatisfactory performance on a job), but LGBTQ people have *additional* risk: they may be fired from a job because of anti-LGBTQ discrimination.

Keeping all else equal, one would hypothesize that the LGBTQ person will experience more job losses, which explains excess stress and related disorders, compared with the cisgender straight person.

Figure 6.1 depicts the model showing that health outcomes (in the box marked i) are caused by stressors (c, d, f) related to disadvantaged social position (b), which is embedded in social environment. In my work I have described different stress processes, including stressful events (such as job loss described above), as well as more *proximal* processes, which are stressors that work through the internalization of social processes. The proximal processes include internalized homophobia, expectations of rejection and discrimination in social interactions, and hiding or nondisclosure of one's sexual identity for fear of being singled out for discrimination and prejudice. Like all stress processes, minority stress describes coping and social support (h) as resilience factors that also can be described as related to individual or social environmental processes (Meyer 2015). These processes ameliorate the impact of stress on health outcomes, so that the greater the effective support and coping, the fewer adverse outcomes resulting from stress. Thus, health outcomes are determined by the total effect of stress, coping, and

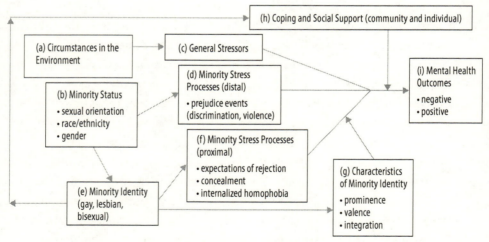

Figure 6.1. The minority stress model, showing minority stress processes in the relationship between disadvantaged social statuses and health. From Meyer 2003. Copyright © 2003 American Psychological Association

social support. Identity (e) and characteristics of identity (g), such as whether an LGB person views their identity as positive or negative, can interact with stress processes to moderate the impact of stress. Identity (e) is also a mediator that can lead to greater resilience by, for example, leading to stronger affiliation with the LGBTQ community and, thus, greater coping and support (Frost and Meyer 2012; Kertzner, Meyer, Frost, and Stirratt 2009).

From Theory to Research

For a theory to guide research and intervention, it has to direct us to research methods and measures. There are many approaches to the study of minority stress. *Between-group* studies that compare LGBTQ populations with heterosexual cisgender populations most directly test health disparities. Of course, studies could focus on various subpopulations—transgender vs. cisgender, lesbian/bisexual women vs. heterosexual women, etc.—but to directly assess health disparities, two populations are compared with one presumed to be the disadvantaged (that is, the population is subject to prejudice and stigma) and the other more advantaged, everything else held constant. Thus, the hypotheses could be tested that (a) the disadvantaged (i.e., LGBTQ) population is exposed to more stress than the advantaged (i.e., heterosexual cisgender) population; (b) the disadvantaged population has more disorder or distress; and (c) stress processes explain the excess disorder—that is, stress mediates the relationship between disadvantaged status and disorder.

A *within-group* study design focuses on one sample of the LGBTQ population or subgroups within the LGBTQ populations. In within-group designs, the researcher examines predictors of various levels of exposure to minority stress but, unlike between-groups studies, a within-group study does not directly assess health disparities. (The interested reader can read more about within- versus between-groups design at Schwartz and Meyer 2010.) Thus, within-group studies have described the workings of minority stress among LGBTQ populations and its impact on health. For example, a study could show variations in exposure to stress and support and their associations with various health outcomes. Other study designs may look at ecological differences. One example of this is comparing LGBTQ people residing in regions where prejudice and stigma are high with those residing in regions with lower levels of prejudice and stigma. This would demonstrate the impact of reduction in levels of prejudice and stigma on health—for example, that suicide ideation would be less prevalent among sexual minority youth in regions where there is greater social acceptance for LGBTQ youth (Hatzenbuheler 2011).

Theory to Research Example: The Generations Study

As an example, I now describe a recently funded study that uses minority stress theory to assess generational changes in the experience of minority stress (grant R01HD078526). I use excerpts from a National Institutes of Health (NIH) grant application to give the reader some concrete examples of components of a research proposal. The premise of the study is that the changing social environment has impacted LGB people differently depending on when they came of age and the kind of social environment they absorbed as children and throughout their lifespan. More about the study, its investigators, and progress can be reviewed at www.generations-study.com. The Generations study focuses on sexual minorities; a sister study, www.transpop.org, focuses on transgender individuals. We study these populations in two separate studies because the issues and related study questions and methods that were central to our hypotheses in the two studies were significantly different.

The Generations investigators proposed a longitudinal design to compare three cohorts of LGB individuals—ages 18–25, 34–41, and 51–59—who are distinct in that they were exposed to significantly different social environments when they came of age. The study concerns ways that minority stress predicts a range of health outcomes similarly or differently across the three cohorts. The study uses a mixed-methods design that allows the investigators to gain knowledge from both qualitative and survey data, where each source of data provides insight into the questions under study. For the survey, the investigators used an innovative procedure to recruit a sample representative of US Black,

Latino, and White LGB people and assess them at baseline and annually for three years thereafter. For the qualitative assessment, the investigators used a narrative life history approach to assess a diverse group of Black, Latino, White, and Asian LGB individuals in urban and rural regions of New York, California, and Arizona (Frost et al. unpublished).

To bring about a study with complex questions, collaboration among a team of researchers with diverse expertise and experience is required. In addition to myself, the investigators are Dr. Stephen Russell, a sociologist in life-course studies who has been studying the health and well-being of LGB youth, documenting significant health risk among sexual minority adolescents (Russell and Joyner 2001; Russell, Driscoll, and Truong, 2002; Russell and Consolacion, 2003); Dr. Marguerita Lightfoot, whose expertise is in health promotion with work on the development of health-promotion interventions for ethnically diverse LGB populations; Dr. David Frost, who has expertise in the qualitative and quantitative methods proposed in the study (Frost 2011a; Frost and Meyer 2009; 2012) and has published widely on the health and well-being of LGB populations (Frost 2011b); Dr. Phillip Hammack, who has contributed to theoretical perspectives on sexual identity development that emphasize life-course development (Hammack 2005) and narrative (Hammack and Cohler 2009) and has studied historical and political context and identity development in LGB youth (Hammack and Cohler 2011; Hammack, Thompson, and Pilecki 2009); and Dr. Bianca Wilson, who brings expertise in multimethod research—for example, using intersectionality perspective, she studied how social norms, culture, oppression, and community settings affect ethnic and sexual minorities' health and health care. Finally, Dr. Mark Handcock, a statistician, contributes with expertise focusing on the development of statistical models for the analysis of social network data, spatial processes, longitudinal data, and the combination of survey and population-level information. In addition to these investigators, a team of scientific advisors provided additional guidance in understanding aging in LGB populations, lesbian health, relationships and marriage, LGB Latino/Latina issues, including immigration and acculturation, and other issues.

Merging of Minority Stress and Other Theoretical Approaches

The Generations study was based on the investigators' understanding of health disparities as likely to emerge during times of salient life transitions (Pearlin, Schieman, Fazio, and Meersman 2005; Halfon and Hochstein 2002). The LGB life course is characterized by some transitions distinct to LGBs, such as awareness of LGB identity and coming out (Hamilton and Mahalik 2009) as well as normative life transitions, such as establishing healthy adult relationships, completing education, and beginning employment (Arnett 2000).

Because of the vast and relatively quick changes in the status of homosexuality in our society over the past 50 years (Loftus 2001; Tucker 2006; Baunach 2012), recent cohorts of LGBs have faced different environments in terms of legal status, community attitudes, and parental and familial acceptance. Such shifts in the social environment of LGBs change the characteristics of minority stress and its impact on health. For example, a social environment that is more affirming of LGB identities in some regions of the United States is related to lower psychiatric morbidity and suicide (Hatzenbuehler 2001; Hatzenbuehler, Keyes, and Hasin, 2009; Hatzenbuehler, Keyes, and McLaughlin 2011). We do not know, however, how minority stress has changed for different cohorts of LGBs (if it has at all). For example, internalized homophobia is a minority stressor that is a significant predictor of adverse health and well-being (Frost and Meyer 2009). But has greater social acceptance of LGBs lessened internalized homophobia and its negative impact among today's LGB youth compared with earlier cohorts? Similarly, LGBs in older cohorts often experienced rejection or some degree of alienation from heterosexual family. Have improved social attitudes changed older LGB people's relationships with, and level of support from, family members? Answers to these questions are important in understanding the causes of health disparities, in developing public health and policy interventions, and in improving clinical interventions with LGBs across the life course. Therefore, the Generations study attempts to answer such questions by assessing similarities and differences in trajectories of the experience of minority stress, resilience, and health in three cohorts of LGB individuals who came of age during three distinct historical periods with immense implications for LGB life.

Just as experiences of stress and resilience depend on one's social environment across the lifespan, notions about identity also vary. Our knowledge of identity development of LGB people is based on research conducted in a context where societal conditions were markedly different and more unfavorable to LGB people than today (Cass 1979; Coleman 1982). These identity-development models have been criticized, but little empirical evidence exists to assist in revising them (Eliason and Schope 2007). Thus, we know little about how today's LGB youth's identity development conforms to or challenges established knowledge of sexual identity (Wilson and Harper 2012; Hammack and Cohler 2009). The Generations study investigators assess similarities and differences in trajectories of LGB identity across the three cohorts. In addition, traditional identity models, especially coming-out models of the 1970s and 1980s, have focused primarily on the experience of White LGBs. In Generations, the investigators explore differences in identity at the intersection of multiple identities related to both structural (e.g., gender, race/ethnicity, social class, residential area) and cultural (e.g., gender expression, religiosity) dimensions of social status. Also, significantly, most—if not all—research on identity development has come from nonprobability samples, which tend to select LGBs who are most likely to participate in mainstream LGB institutions and, thus, are more likely to identify as LGB (Meyer and Colten 1999; Meyer and Wilson 2009). This is a limitation that the Generations study's reliance on a probability sample comes to address.

Intersections of Gender and Race/Ethnicity

Stress, coping, social support, and identity are all affected by one's social statuses in addition to sexual orientation. Gender and racial/ethnic differences in identity and health among LGBs are a function of exposure to multiple forms of oppression and access to support services in LGBTQ community settings (Meyer, Schwartz, and Frost 2008). The Generations study contributes to knowledge about how intersections of race/ethnicity and gender influence conceptualizations of sexual identity, experiences with minority stress, health outcomes, and health care utilization across the lifespan. Oversampling of Black and Latino LGBs in a national probability sample is an especially important aspect of the study because it ensures power for analysis by these intersections.

Intervention and Health Care Service Utilization

Social and health services targeting LGB people have traditionally been implemented through LGB-identified service delivery (e.g., an LGBTQ community center). This approach is based on the premise that LGBs will seek to affiliate with LGB organizations and service providers because they offer support and affirmation and because LGBs fear that they may be stigmatized by non-LGB providers who are not culturally competent to provide LGB health services. It is possible, given changes in social stigma over time, and changes in minority stress, identity, and affiliation patterns, that today's LGBs may not seek LGB-identified health services to the same extent as earlier cohorts. Generations study investigators assess health care utilization patterns, noting differences and similarities among subgroups of LGBs (e.g., by race/ethnicity). The investigators hypothesized that the strength and nature of LGB identity and other cultural and structural social dimensions (e.g., race/ethnicity, rural residence) will be related to affiliation with the community and utilization of services in the LGBTQ community (Coker, Austin, and Schuster 2010). Knowledge gained from this study will inform public health planning and intervention design that can target various subgroups of LGBs.

Generations Study Hypotheses

Consistent with the goal of the study, the investigators have four main aims in assessing cohort-related differences in the experience of minority stress. In Aim 1 the investigators described identity trajectories. They hypothesized that younger cohorts differ from older cohorts in that their LGB identity would be less central, and they would be less strongly identified with an LGBTQ community, have a younger average age of coming out, and have different understandings of sexual orientation and identity. In terms of intersectionality, the investigators hypothesized that older White gay and bisexual men would be more likely than other LGBs to conceptualize their sexual identities independent of their race and gender identities.

In Aim 2, the investigators described patterns of stress and resilience, hypothesizing that there are differences in the patterns of exposure to minority stress related to cohort and age. Thus, the researchers hypothesized, younger LGB people would experience more prejudice (e.g., bullying while at school) than did older LGB people, but younger LGB people would have less internalized homophobia than older LGB people. In terms of resilience, the researchers hypothesized that members of older cohorts would have greater connection and affiliation with the LGBTQ community and greater social support from other LGBTQ people than members of younger cohorts. At the same time, it was hypothesized, while younger LGB people would have fewer LGBTQ connections and support, they would have greater support from heterosexual family and friends because of greater acceptance of LGB people in society today. The investigators again explore differences by intersectional identities defined by gender, race/ethnicity, class, and geographic region. For example, they hypothesized that because of the additive burden of prejudice related to their race/ethnicity, racial/ethnic minority LGB people will experience more stress and will rely on coping strategies to negotiate both race/ethnic and sexual identity stress.

In Aim 3 the investigators describe patterns of health care utilization. They hypothesized that the younger cohort of LGBs would be less connected to LGBTQ-identified public health and social services, or view them as less central for receiving health services, and more likely than older cohorts of LGB to utilize services that are not LGBTQ-identified. In terms of intersection, the investigators posited various hypotheses—e.g., that racial/ethnic minority lesbians would be less likely than gay and bisexual men of all race/ethnicities to access LGBTQ-identified public health services because of the greater reliance of gay and bisexual men on HIV/AIDS-related services located at LGBTQ organizations.

Finally, in Aim 4, the investigators assess similarities and differences in how minority stress (including stressors, coping, and social support) affects a range of adverse health outcomes (mental and physical health, health behaviors, and health care utilization) in younger versus older LGB cohorts. They hypothesized that the minority stress model would predict health outcomes in the younger and older cohorts, but that pathways to outcomes will differ among the cohorts in accordance with findings in Aims 1 and 2.

Methods and Measures

A review of the Generations methods is beyond the scope of this chapter, but I want to share some insight about measures. I am sometimes asked which measure I use to study minority stress. The answer, of course, is that there is no one measure of minority stress. The minority stress model does not lend itself to one measure because it comprises many constructs related to its origin in various theories. To demonstrate how investigators address this, the measures that were proposed for the Generations study are summarized in table 6.1. The Generations study, as described above, uses minority stress theory to build hypotheses about differences and similarities among three cohorts of LGB people, but it also uses other theories such as intersectionality and lifespan. Therefore, the measures selected by the investigators represent a variety of constructs that represent concepts raised by these theories

Finally, I briefly cite one of the analytic approaches and measures the Generations investigators use. For example, to assess the stress → outcome relationships described in Aim 4, the investigators will fit components of the conceptual model (fig. 6.1) to the data using Structural Equation Modeling (SEM) and examine standard criteria for indicators of model fit (Chi-Square, CFI, RMSEA). This will allow for tests of the implied causal, mediating, and moderating processes specified in the model.

Conclusions

The Generations study is a good example of how minority stress theory can be tested in a research project. The study is an example of a within-group design because there is no heterosexual comparison group against

Table 6.1 Measures Proposed for the Generations Study

Classification	Measure	Study Instruments
Health Outcomes	Center for Epidemiologic Studies Depression Scale	Twenty items self-report depressive symptoms scale for research in the general population (Radloff 1977). The scale has been used in numerous studies including studies with diverse LGB populations.
	WMH-CIDI suicidality	Seven items inquire about lifetime suicide ideation, planning, and attempt; four additional items inquire about intent and severity of attempt among those with an attempt (Kessler and Ustun 2004).
	Physical health	SF-12 (Short Form-12 Health Survey), a twelve-item widely used measure of physical and mental health (Ware, Kosinski, Turner-Bowker, and Gandek 2002).
	Social well-being	Fifteen-item social well-being scale has five subscales: social acceptance, social actualization, social contribution, social coherence, and social integration (Keyes 1998).
	Health-related quality of life	Three items from the Centers for Disease Control and Prevention 2011 Behavioral Risk Factor Surveillance System (BRFSS), a state-based system of health surveys with over 350,000 interviews a year that collects information on health risk behaviors, preventive health practices, and health care access primarily related to chronic disease and injury (CDC 2011).
	Alcohol consumption	Four items from the CDC's 2011 BRFSS assessing the frequency and amount of alcohol consumed over the past 30 days, including the frequency of binge drinking (CDC 2011).
	Tobacco use	Five items from the CDC's 2011 BRFSS assessing use of tobacco products, including cigarettes, chewing tobacco, and smokeless tobacco. One item assesses whether a respondent has tried to quit smoking within the past year (CDC 2011).
	Utilization of health care	Four items from the CDC's 2011 BRFSS assessing whether a respondent has health insurance coverage, has a primary care provider, or for financial reasons has not been able to seek necessary healthcare. The final item assesses time since last routine check-up (CDC 2011). For each provider, respondent is asked whether this primarily an LGBT provider.
	Consumption of fruits and vegetables	Six items from the CDC's 2011 BRFSS that capture the frequency of fruit and vegetable consumption over the past 30 days (CDC 2011).
	Physical activity	Eight items from the CDC's 2011 BRFSS that assess the frequency, duration, and types of physical activity engaged in over the past 30 days, excluding the time spent at a regular job (CDC 2011).

(*continued*)

Table 6.1 (Continued)

Classification	Measure	Study Instruments
Stressors	Conceal sexual identity ("Out")	Five items asking about degree of sexual orientation outness to: family, straight friends, LGB friends, co-workers, and health care providers (Meyer, Rossano, Ellis, and Bradford 2002).
	Perception of stigma	Six-item measure of perceiving stigma related to one's race/ethnicity, gender, sexual identity, and class (Link 1987).
	Internalized homophobia	Eight-item scale modified from one developed by Martin and Dean (1987) and used in many studies (Herek, Cogan, Gillis, and Glunt 1998; Frost and Meyer 2009).
	Stressful life events and perceived stress	Fourteen items—the Alcohol Use Disorder and Associated Disabilities Interview Schedule-IV (AUDADIS-IV) events in past year (e.g., being fired or laid off from a job) (Ruan, Goldstein, Chou, Smith, Saha, Pickering, et al. 2008).
	Chronic strains	Twenty-eight-item scale based on Wheaton's conceptualization and Turner et al.'s elaboration (Wheaton, 1999), Turner & Avison, 2003). Participants asked to indicate how true statements are about their life presently (13 subscales covering 13 areas of life such as relationships, loneliness, and caretaking responsibilities) (Turner and Avison 2003).
	Experience of discrimination	Eight items assess frequency of day-to-day discrimination and whether discrimination was related to gender, race/ethnicity, physical appearance, gender nonconformity, sexual orientation, or handicap (Dressler, Oths, and Gravlee 2005; Williams, Yu, Jackson, and Anderson 1997).
Identity	Coming-out milestones	Seven items calculating the age when a respondent first realized his/her sexual identity and subsequently disclosed his/her identity to family and friends (e.g., age at interview minus age of first realization) (Durso and Meyer 2013).
	Identity salience	Three items asking respondents to nominate race/ethnic, sexual orientation and other identities, roles, or traits to describe themselves as well as rank their relative importance (Thoit 1995).
	Multigroup Ethnic Identity Measure Revised (MEIM-R)	Six-item measure of ethnic group commitment and exploration (Phinney and Ong 2007)
Resilience / Coping and Social Support	Mastery	Seven-item measure of feeling of control and agency over life circumstances (Pearlin and Schooler 1978).
	Brief resilience	Six-item measure of the ability to bounce back or recover from stress (Smith, Dalen, Wiggins, Tooley, Christopher, and Bernard 2008).

Classification	Measure	Study Instruments
	Social support matrix	Instrument assessing the composition of social support networks and types of support received (Fisher 1977).
	Behavioral affiliation with the LGBT community	Nine-item inventory of participation in and/or attendance at organizations and activities (Mills, Stall, Pollack, Paul, Binson, Canchola et al. 2001)
	Connectedness to the LGBT community	Eight items assessing the degree of closeness to the LGBT community as well as the quality of connections (Saewyc 2011).
Structural and Cultural Dimensions of Social Statuses		
	Demographics	A range of demographic background information including sexual orientation and identity, race/ethnicity, gender, relationship status, and children.
	Social class	Education measured as highest education level attained. Per capita debt to asset ratio calculated as the sum of total household liabilities and total assets, divided by number of adults in household (Conger, Wallace, Sun, Simmons, McLoyd, and Brody 2002).
	Machismo/masculinity	Twenty-item measure of traditional *machismo* (e.g., aggressiveness) and positive aspects of *caballerismo* (e.g., ethnic affiliation) (Arciniega, Anderson, Tovar-Blank, and Tracey 2008).
	Gender conformity and expression	Seven-item measure on levels of childhood gender conformity (Wylie, Corliss, Prokop, and Austin 2010).
	Acculturation	Twelve-item measure assessing three factors: language use, media, and ethnic social relations (Marin, Sabogal, Marin, Otero-Sabogal, and Perez-Stable 1987).
	Religiosity	Six-item measure adapted from the Brief Multidimensional Measure of Religiousness/Spirituality (Fetzer Institute and National Institute on Aging Workgroup 1999).
	Place of residence	One item asking about current hometown zip code to be recoded as per the US Census residential region as well to distinguish as rural vs. urban.

which health disparities can be assessed. However, the study's aims demonstrate that components of the model can be tested in various groups within the LGB population based on, for example, age, gender, and race/ethnicity. The Generations study is also a test of components of the minority stress model. It assesses whether all minority stress components are relevant across the three cohorts under study. In that sense, the model can be updated based on Generations research findings. For example, if the hypothesis that young LGB people no longer suffer from internalized homophobia is supported, then the model may need to be updated by removing the role of internalized homophobia as a stressor that predicts health outcomes (at least for young LGB people). That internalized homophobia ceased to play a role in the development of LGB people seems unlikely to me at present (research findings will show us whether this hypothesis is supported or not). But perhaps it is plausible sometime in the future, as social attitudes and conditions regarding LGB people continue to improve. The important lesson here is that the model is to be tested and findings, to the extent that they are consistent and convincing, could lead to updating the model.

The model can also be expanded to incorporate new theories. For example, Hatzenbuehler (2009) suggested that internal psychological processes—including emotional dysregulation, social/interpersonal problems, and cognitive processes—are mediators that connect minority stress to risk for psychopathology. This expands the model to incorporate both the social conditions and the more psychological processes. Other expansions can lead to the study of pathophysiological pathways on one hand (Juster et al. 2015) and, on the other hand, to understanding structures that initiate minority stress processes (Hatzenbuehler, Keyes, and Hasin 2009).

Expanding minority stress to intervention would require new research, including identifying specific areas for intervention along the minority stress model (Meyer and Frost 2013). Combining minority stress and syndemic work, as described by Stall and colleagues (Stall et al. 2003; Herrick et al. 2013), would enrich both theories as investigators seek to identify fundamental causes associated with stigma that can impact syndemic production (Hatzenbuehler, Phelan, and Link 2013).

Finally, minority stress can be articulated for populations and subpopulations as more specific stress processes are added to the model (or unhelpful ones deducted). As noted above, a model of minority stress was adopted for transgender individuals by Hendricks and Testa (2012) and Testa et al. (2015). The authors highlighted gender affirmation—

"the process by which individuals are affirmed in their gender identity through social interactions" (Sevelius 2013, 675)—as a particularly important stressor in the lives of transgender people.

Theories in general, and the minority stress theory specifically, can be used to inform us by directing research and intervention to gain new knowledge. As social conditions that affect the health of LGBTQ people change, researchers need to examine their models and change them, when necessary, based on evidence. Studying socially embedded health and well-being requires us to continue to test, update, and expand our framework for understanding health and health disparities in sexual and gender minorities.

References

Allport, G. W. 1954. *The Nature of Prejudice*. Cambridge, MA: Addison-Wesley Publication Company.

Arciniega, G. M., Anderson, T. C., Tovar-Blank, Z. G., and Tracey, T. J. 2008. Toward a fuller conception of machismo: Development of a traditional machismo and caballerismo scale. *Journal of Counseling Psychology* 55(1): 19–33.

Arnett, J. J. 2000. Emerging adulthood: A theory of development from the late teens through the twenties. *American Psychologist* 55(5): 469–80.

Baunach, M. 2012. Changing same-sex marriage attitudes in America from 1988 through 2010. *Public Opinion Quarterly* 76(2): 364–78.

Bayer, R. 1981. *Homosexuality and American Psychiatry*. New York: Basic Books.

Bockting, W. O., Miner, M. H., Swinburne Romine, R. E., Hamilton, A., and Coleman, E. 2013. Stigma, mental health, and resilience in an online sample of the US transgender population. *American Journal of Public Health* 103(5): 943–51

Bockting, W. O., Coleman, E., Deutsch, M. B., Guillamon, A., Meyer, I., Meyer, W. . . . and Ettner, R. 2016. Adult development and quality of life of transgender and gender nonconforming people. *Current Opinion in Endocrinology, Diabetes and Obesity* 23(2): 188–97.

Cass, V. C. 1979. Homosexual identity formation: A theoretical model. *Journal of Homosexuality* 4(3): 219–35.

Centers for Disease Control and Prevention (CDC). 2011. *Behavioral Risk Factor Surveillance System Survey Questionnaire*. Atlanta, GA: US Department of Health and Human Services, Centers for Disease Control and Prevention.

Cochran, S. D. 2001. Emerging issues in research on lesbians' and gay men's mental health: Does sexual orientation really matter? *American Psychologist* 56: 931–47.

Cochran, S. D., and Mays, V. M. 2000a. Lifetime prevalence of suicide symptoms and affective disorders among men reporting same-sex sexual partners: Results from NHANES III. *American Journal of Public Health* 90: 573–78.

Cochran, S. D., and Mays, V. M. 2000b. Relation between psychiatric syndromes and behaviorally defined sexual orientation in a sample of the US population. *American Journal of Epidemiology* 151: 516–23.

Coker, T. R., Austin, S. B., and Schuster, M. A. 2010. The health and health care of lesbian, gay, and bisexual adolescents. *Annual Review of Public Health* 31: 457–77.

Coleman, E. 1982. Developmental stages of the coming out process. *Journal of Homosexuality* 7(2–3): 31–43.

Conger, R. D., Wallace, L. E., Sun, Y., Simmons, R. L., McLoyd, V. C., and Brody, G. H. 2002. Economic pressure in African American families: A replication and extension of the family stress model. *Developmental Psychology* 38(2): 179–93.

Dohrenwend, B. P. 1998. *Adversity, Stress, and Psychopathology.* New York: Oxford University Press.

Dressler, W. W., Oths, K. S., and Gravlee, C. C. 2005. Race and ethnicity in public health research: Models to explain health disparities. *Annual Review of Anthropology* 34: 231–252.

Durso, L. E., and Meyer, I. H. 2013. Patterns and predictors of disclosure of sexual orientation to healthcare providers among lesbians, gay men, and bisexuals. *Sexuality Research and Social Policy* 10(1): 35–42.

Eliason, M. J., and Schope, R. 2007. Shifting sands or solid foundation? Lesbian, gay, bisexual, and transgender identity formation. In I. Meyer and M. E. Northridge, eds., *The Health of Sexual Minorities,* 3–26. New York: Springer.

Fergusson, D. M., Horwood, L. J. and Beautrais, A. L. 1999. Is sexual orientation related to mental health problems and suicidality in young people? *Archives of General Psychiatry* 56(10): 876–80.

Fetzer Institute and National Institute on Aging Workgroup. 1999. *Multidimensional Measurement of Religiousness/Spirituality for Use in Health Research.* Kalamazoo, MI: Fetzer Institute.

Fisher, C. S. 1977. Networking analysis and urban studies. In C. S. Fisher et al., eds. *Networks and Places: Social Relations in the Urban Setting,* 19–37. New York: Free Press.

Frost, D. M. 2011a. Stigma and intimacy in same-sex relationships: A narrative approach. *Journal of Family Psychology* 25(1): 1–10.

Frost, D. M. 2011b. Social stigma and its consequences for the socially stigmatized. *Social and Personality Psychology Compass* 5(11): 824–39.

Frost, D. M., Hammack, P. L., Wilson, B. D. M., Russell, S. T., Lightfoot, M., and Meyer, I. H. (Unpublished manuscript). A qualitative approach to understanding minority stress, identity, and health in the context of social change.

Frost, D. M., and Meyer, I. H. 2009. Internalized homophobia and relationship quality among lesbians, gay men, and bisexuals. *Journal of Counseling Psychology* 56(1): 97–109.

Frost, D. M., and Meyer, I. H. 2012. Measuring community connectedness among diverse sexual minority populations. *Journal of Sex Research* 48(1), 36–49.

Goffman, E. 1963. *Stigma: Notes on the Management of Spoiled Identity.* Englewood Cliffs, NJ: Prentice-Hall.

Gordon, A., and Meyer, I. H. 2007. Gender nonconformity as a target of prejudice, discrimination and violence against LGB individuals. *Journal of LGBT Health Research* 3(3): 55–71.

Halfon, N., and Hochstein, M. 2002. Life course health development: An integrated framework for developing health, policy, and research. *Milbank Quarterly* 80(3): 433–79.

Hamilton, C. J., and Mahalik, J. R. 2009. Minority stress, masculinity, and social norms predicting gay men's health risk behaviors. *Journal of Counseling Psychology* 56(1): 132–41.

Hammack, P. L. 2005. The life course development of human sexual orientation: An integrative paradigm. *Human Development* 48(5): 267–90.

Hammack, P. L., and Cohler, B. J. 2009. Narrative engagement and sexual identity: An interdisciplinary approach to the study of sexual lives. In P. L. Hammack and B. J. Cohler, eds., *The Story of Sexual Identity: Narrative Perspectives on the Gay and Lesbian Life Course*, 3–22. New York: Oxford University Press.

Hammack, P. L., and Cohler, B. J. 2011. Narrative, identity, and the politics of exclusion: Social change and the gay and lesbian life course. *Sexuality Research and Social Policy* 8: 162–82.

Hammack, P. L., Thompson E. M., and Pilecki, A. 2009. Configurations of identity among sexual minority youth: Context, desire, and narrative. *Journal of Youth and Adolescence* 38(7): 867–83.

Hatzenbuehler, M. L. 2009. How does sexual minority stigma "get under the skin"? A psychological mediation framework. *Psychological Bulletin* 135(5): 707–30

Hatzenbuehler, M. L. 2011. The social environment and suicide attempts in lesbian, gay, and bisexual youth. *Pediatrics* 127(5): 896–903.

Hatzenbuehler, M. L., Keyes, K. M., and Hasin D. S. 2009. State-level policies and psychiatric morbidity in lesbian, gay, and bisexual populations. *American Journal of Public Health* 99(12): 2275–81.

Hatzenbuehler, M. L., Keyes, K. M., and McLaughlin, K. A. 2011. The protective effects of social/contextual factors on psychiatric morbidity in LGB populations. *International Journal of Epidemiology* 40(4): 1071–80.

Hendricks, M. L., and Testa, R. J. 2012. A conceptual framework for clinical work with transgender and gender nonconforming clients: An adaptation of Minority Stress Model. *Professional Psychology: Research and Practice* 43(5): 460–67.

Herek, G. M., Cogan, J. C., Gillis, J. R., and Glunt, E. K. 1998. Correlates of internalized homophobia in a community sample of lesbians and gay men. *Journal of the Gay and Lesbian Medical Association* 2:17–25.

Herrell, R., Goldberg, J., True, W. R., Visvanathan, R., Lyons, M., Eisen, S., and Tsuang, M. T. 1999. Sexual orientation and suicidality: A co-twin control study in adult men. *Archives of General Psychiatry* 56(10): 867–74.

Herrick, A. L., Lim, S. H., Plankey, M. W., Chmiel, J. S., Guadamuz, T. T., Kao, U. . . . Stall, R. 2013. Adversity and syndemic production among men participating in the Multicenter AIDS Cohort Study: A life-course approach. *American Journal of Public Health* 103(1): 79–85.

Holmes, T. H., and Rahe, R. H. 1967. The social re-adjustment rating scale. *Journal of Psychosomatic Research* 11: 213–18.

Juster, R., Hatzenbuehler, M. L., Mendrek, A., Pfaus, J. G., Smith, N. G., Johnson, P. J. . . . Pruessner, J. C. 2015. Sexual orientation modulates endocrine stress reactivity. *Biological Psychiatry* 77(7): 668–76.

Kessler, R. C., and Ustun, T. B. 2004. The World Mental Health (WMH) survey initiative version of the World Health Organization (WHO) composite international diagnostic interview (CIDI). *International Journal of Methods Psychiatry Research* 13(2): 93–121.

Kertzner, R. M., Meyer, I. H., Frost, D. M., and Stirratt, M. J. 2009. Psychological well-being in middle-aged and older gay men. In D. Herdt and B. de Vries, eds., *Gay and Lesbian Aging: Research and Future Directions*. New York: Springer.

Keyes, L. M. 1998. Social well-being. *Social Psychology Quarterly* 61(2): 121–40.

Lazarus, R. S., and Folkman, S. 1984. *Stress, Appraisal, and Coping*. New York: Springer.

Lewin, K. 1952. *Field Theory in Social Science: Selected Theoretical Papers by Kurt Lewin*. London: Tavistock.

Link, B. G. 1987. Understanding labeling effects in the area of mental disorders: An assessment of the effects of expectations of rejection. *American Sociological Review* 52(1): 96–112.

Link, B. G., and Phelan, J. 1995. Social conditions as fundamental causes of disease. *Journal of Health and Social Behavior* (extra issue): 80–94.

Loftus, J. 2001. America's liberalization in attitudes toward homosexuality, 1973 to 1998. *American Sociological Review* 66(5): 762–82.

Marin, G., Sabogal, F., Marin, V., Otero-Sabogal, R., and Perez-Stable, J. 1987. Development of a short acculturation scale for Hispanics. *Hispanic Journal of Behavioral Sciences* 9(2): 183–205.

Marmor, J. 1980. Epilogue: Homosexuality and the issue of mental illness. In J. Marmor ed., *Homosexual Behavior: A Modern Reappraisal*, 391–401. New York: Basic Books.

Martin, J. L., and Dean, L. 1987. Summary of measures: Mental health effects of AIDS on at-risk homosexual men. Unpublished work.

Malyon, A. K. 1982. Psychotherapeutic implications of internalized homophobia in gay men. *Journal of Homosexuality* 7(2–3): 59–69.

Mays, V. M., and Cochran, S. D. 2001. Mental health correlates of perceived discrimination among lesbian, gay, and bisexual adults in the United States. *American Journal of Public Health* 91: 1869–76.

Meyer, I. H. 1995. Minority stress and mental health in gay men. *Journal of Health and Social Behavior* 36: 38–56.

Meyer, I. H. 2003. Prejudice, social stress, and mental health in lesbian, gay, and bisexual populations: Conceptual issues and research evidence. *Psychological Bulletin* 129(5): 674–97.

Meyer, I. H. 2015. Resilience in the study of minority stress and health of sexual and gender minorities. *Psychology of Sexual Orientation and Gender Diversity* 2(3): 209–13.

Meyer, I. H., and Colten, M. E. 1999. Sampling gay men: Random digit dialing versus sources in the gay community. *Journal of Homosexuality* 37(4): 99–110.

Meyer, I. H., and Frost, D. M. 2013. Minority stress and the health of sexual minorities. In C. J. Patterson and A. R. D'Augelli, eds., *Handbook of Psychology and Sexual Orientation*, 252–66. New York: Oxford University Press.

Meyer I. H., Rossano, L., Ellis, J., and Bradford, J. 2002. A brief telephone interview to identify lesbian and bisexual women in random digit dialing sampling. *Journal of Sex Research* 39(2): 139–44.

Meyer, I. H., Schwartz, S., and Frost, D. M. 2008. Social patterning of stress and coping: Does disadvantaged social statuses confer more stress and fewer coping resources? *Social Science Medicine* 67(3): 368–79.

Meyer, I. H., and Wilson, P. A. 2009. Sampling lesbian, gay, and bisexual populations. *Journal of Counseling Psychology* 56(1): 23–31.

Mills, T. C., Stall, R., Pollack, L., Paul, J. P., Binson, D., Canchola, J., and Catania, J. A. 2001. Health-related characteristics of men who have sex with men: A comparison of those living in "gay ghettos" with those living elsewhere. *American Journal of Public Health* 91(6): 980–83.

Pearlin, L. I. 1982. The social context of stress. In L. Goldberger and S. Breznitz, eds., *Handbook of Stress: Theoretical and Clinical Aspects*, 367–79. New York: Academic Press.

Pearlin, L. I., Schieman, S., Fazio, E. M., and Meersman, S. C. 2005. Stress, health, and the life course: Some conceptual perspectives. *Journal of Health and Social Behavior* 46(2): 205–19.

Pearlin, L.I., and Schooler, C. 1978. The structure of coping. *Journal of Health and Social Behavior* 19(1): 2–21.

Phinney, J. S., and Ong, A. D. 2007. Conceptualization and measurement of ethnic identity: Current status and future directions. *Journal of Counseling Psychology* 54(3): 271–81.

Radloff, L. S. 1977. The CES-D Scale: A self-report depression scale for research in the general population. *Applied Psychological Measures* 1(3): 385–401.

Robins L. N., and Regier, D. A., eds. 1991. *Psychiatric Disorders in America: The Epidemiologic Catchment Area Study*. New York: Free Press.

Ruan, W. J., Goldstein, R. B., Chou, S. P., Smith, S. M., Saha, T. D., Pickering, R. P., Dawson, D., Huang, B., Stinson, F. S., and Grant, B. F. 2008. The alcohol use disorder and associated disabilities interview schedule-IV (AUDADIS-IV): Reliability of new psychiatric diagnostic modules and risk factors in a general population sample. *Drug and Alcohol Dependence* 92(1–3): 27–36.

Russell, S. T., and Joyner, K. 2001. Adolescent sexual orientation and suicide risk: Evidence from a national study. *American Journal of Public Health* 91(8): 1276–81

Russell, S. T., Driscoll, A. K., and Truong, N. 2002. Adolescent same-sex romantic attractions and relationships: Implications for substance use and abuse. *American Journal of Public Health* 92(2): 198–202.

Russell, S. T., and Consolacion, T. B. 2003. Adolescent romance and emotional health in the United States: Beyond binaries. *Journal of Clinical Child and Adolescent Psychology* 32(4): 499–508.

Saewyc, E. M. 2011. Research on adolescent sexual orientation: Development, health disparities, stigma, and resilience. *Journal of Research on Adolescence* 21(1): 256–72.

Sandfort, T. G., de Graaf, R., Bijl, R. V., and Schnabel, P. 2001. Same-sex sexual behavior and psychiatric disorders: Findings from the Netherlands Mental Health Survey and Incidence Study (NEMESIS). *Archives of General Psychiatry* 58: 85–91.

Schwartz, S., and Meyer, I. H. 2010. Mental health disparities research: The impact of within- and between-group analyses on tests of social stress hypotheses. *Social Science and Medicine* 70(8), 1111–18.

Sevelius, J. M. 2013. Gender affirmation: A framework for conceptualizing risk behavior among transgender women of color. *Sex Roles* 68: 11–12.

Smith, B. W., Dalen, J., Wiggins, K., Tooley, E., Christopher, P., and Bernard J. 2008. The brief resilience scale: Assessing the ability to bounce back. *International Journal of Behavioral Medicine* 15(3): 194–200.

Stall, R., Mill, T. C., Williamson, J., Hart, T., Greenwood, G., Paul, J. . . . Catania, J. Q. 2003. Association of co-occurring psychosocial health problems and increased vulnerability to HIV/AIDS among urban men who have sex with men. *American Journal of Public Health* 93(6): 939–42.

Testa, R. J., Habarth, J., Peta, J., Balsam, K., and Bockting, W. 2015. Development of the Gender Minority Stress and Resilience Measure. *Psychology of Sexual Orientation and Gender Diversity* 2(1): 65–77.

Thoits, P. A. 1995. Identity-relevant events and psychological symptoms: A cautionary tale. *Journal of Health and Social Behavior* 36(1): 72–82.

Tucker, W. 2006. Changing heterosexuals' attitudes toward homosexuals: A systematic review of the empirical literature. *Research on Social Work Practice* 16(2): 176–90.

Turner, R. J., and Avison, W. R. 2003. Status variations in stress exposure: Implications for the interpretation of research on race, socioeconomic status, and gender. *Journal of Health and Social Behavior* 44(4): 488–505.

US Department of Health and Human Services. 2000. *Healthy People 2010: Understanding and Improving Health.* 2nd ed. Washington, DC: Government Printing Office.

Vansteenkiste, M., and Sheldon, K. M. 2006. There's nothing more practical than a good theory: Integrating motivational interviewing and self-determination theory. *British Journal of Clinical Psychology* 45: 63–82.

Ware, J. E., Jr., Kosinski, M., Turner-Bowker, D. M., and Gandek, B. 2002. *How to Score Version 2 of the SF-12 Health Survey.* Lincoln, RI: QualityMetric.

Wheaton, B. 1999. The nature of stressors. In A. F. Horwitz and T. L. Scheid, eds., *A Handbook for the Study of Mental Health: Social Contexts, Theories, and Systems,* 176–97. Cambridge: Cambridge University Press.

Williams, D. R., Yu, Y., Jackson, J. S, and Anderson, N. B. 1997. Racial differences in physical and mental health socio-economic status, stress and discrimination. *Journal of Health Psychology* 2(3): 335–51.

Wilson, B. D. M., and Harper, G. 2012. Race and ethnicity in lesbian, gay and bisexual communities. In C. J. Patterson and A. R. D'Augelli, eds., *Handbook of Psychology and Sexual Orientation.* New York: Oxford University Press.

Wylie, S. A., Corliss, H. L., Boulanger, V., Prokop, L. A., and Austin, S. B. 2010. Socially assigned gender nonconformity: A brief measure for use in surveillance and investigation of health disparities. *Sex Roles* 63(3–4): 264–76

SEVEN

Joshua G. Rosenberger

Creating and Adapting LGBTQ-Specific Measures to Explain Disparities

THE 2011 Institute of Medicine report provided the most extensive examination of health issues and disparities among LGBTQ populations, including information on LGBTQ issues across the lifespan, stigma and other barriers to healthcare service, and deficits in LGBTQ health research (Institute of Medicine 2011). The report argued for the need to expand data collection on LGBTQ individuals and to include sexual and gender minorities in all federally funded research; it also highlighted the lack of sufficient data and quality-measurement tools applicable to this research. While the number of tools developed by researchers for use among LGBTQ populations has increased in recent years, they are outstripped by the need for development of new and standardized measures. The simple reasons for this need are either that standardized instruments are not available or that existing tools lack reliability and validity in the settings in which they are being applied.

This chapter highlights how investigators can choose from existing theoretically based variables to measure predictors of health within LGBTQ populations, or if such variables are lacking in the literature, to design and test new measures. The chapter provides a brief overview of some basic concepts in measurement design, describes existing measures appropriate for use with LGBTQ individuals, offers guidelines on how to adapt existing measures, and explains when and how to create entirely new measures. The chapter concludes with a brief description of specific items that should be considered when assessing best practices associated with measuring LGBTQ health. (The measurement of sexual orientation and gender identity is addressed in chapter 4.)

Theory and Utility

Theories consist of "plausible relationships proposed among concepts or sets of concepts" (Strauss and Corbin 1994), and they provide a systematic explanation for the observations that relate to a particular aspect of life (Creswell 1994). A theoretical framework is a critical element of any research study, and the theoretical paradigm that is chosen will provide the foundation for the decision-making related to the types of measures used in a study instrument. A theoretical framework provides scientific justification for investigation, demonstrating that research is not just "made up" but that it is both grounded in and based on scientific theory. Theoretical frameworks guide your research, determining what things you will measure and which statistical relationships you will look for.

Once researchers are at the stage of measurement selection/development, they should have already chosen the theoretical framework on which the study is based. Hundreds of different frameworks have been applied to research with LGBTQ populations. Determining which paradigm is most appropriate for your study typically involves a four-step process that comprises (1) identifying the concepts; (2) identifying interrelationships between concepts; (3) clearly defining concepts; and (4) formulating the theoretical rationale.

A *concept* is an idea that is generalizable such as "risk" or "satisfaction"; once operationalized in a manner in which it can be specifically defined and measured, it is referred to as a *construct*. Through the process of conducting an exhaustive literature review, researchers are able to identify theoretical connections between the variables (i.e., constructs), and a logical theoretical rationale should emerge. When examining the literature, it is useful to look at the theoretical paradigms that have been previously used for studying your particular population, concepts, and constructs. (For an in-depth discussion of the roles and functions of theory in LGBTQ health research, see chapter 6.)

Basic Concepts in Measurement
Conceptualization and Operationalization in Measurement

Conceptualization is the process of specifying a term or concept that researchers want to measure. Conceptualizing can help identify a specific variable to be used or help researchers determine which related behaviors should be observed. *Operationalization* is the process of defining a concept so as to make it clearly distinguishable, measurable, and understandable in terms of empirical observations. Operational definitions must be based on a theory that is generally recognized as valid. The difference between the two is that conceptualization is the process of refining an idea by giving it a very clear, explicit definition; operationalization is the process of linking the conceptual definition with a specific set of measures

Items, Scales, and Indexes

Items, scales, and indexes are tools that are used to measure variables or concepts that are of particular interest. *Scale Development: Theory and Applications* is a standard measurement textbook that can be consulted for detailed guidelines and elements of item development and scale creation, regardless of the study population (DeVellis 2017). Some of the foundational elements of instrument development are briefly summarized below as a base on which LGBTQ measurement challenges can be discussed.

A *single-item measure* attempts to quantify a concept using one question, whereas a *scale* is a cluster of items that are arranged to examine a single dimension of behavior, attitudes, and feelings. Scales can predict outcomes such as behavior, attitudes, and feelings because they measure the underlying traits. Items in a scale used to measure a specific variable such as social support, for example, might include:

1. Do you have someone available to give you good advice about a problem?
2. Do you have someone available to you who shows you love and affection?
3. Do you have someone available to help with daily chores?
4. Do you have someone available to provide you with emotional support?
5. Do you have as much contact as you would like with someone you feel close to, in whom you can trust and confide in?
6. Do you have someone available on whom you can count to listen to you when you need to talk?

Participants would be asked to answer each of these items using Likert scale responses such as "None of the time/All of the time."

Indexes are a more generalized version of a scale; they represent a set of items that contain multiple aspects of interrelated dimensions. Indexes allow for the collapsing of multiple dimensions into a single indicator or score. One such example is the Corporate Equality Index (CEI), a yearly measurement used by the Human Rights Campaign to assess US businesses' commitment to equality in the workplace for LGBTQ employees (Human Rights Campaign 2018). While each business receives a singular score (ranging from 0 to 100), the CEI measures multiple factors associated with equality. The CEI comprises four primary criteria, each with its own subset of dimensions: (1) equal employment opportunity policies; (2) employment benefits; (3) organizational LGBTQ competency; and (4) public commitment. While each of these categories is unique, they are interrelated. The CEI thus provides an overall composite score for each business, allowing for ease of comparison across companies as it relates to LGBTQ equality.

Measurement Scales

Researchers can draw on four scales to measure different variables: (1) a nominal scale, (2) an ordinal scale, (3) an interval scale, and (4) a ratio scale. A *nominal scale* classifies a person or objects into two or more categories. Members of a category have a common set of characteristics, and each member may belong to only one category. Nominal measurement does not take account of relative size; it only represents differences among persons or objects—for example, categorizing someone as LGBTQ or heterosexual. An individual would be classified in either of those categories, but not both. Furthermore, no value is placed on either classification, meaning one person can't be *more* LGBTQ than another person in the same category.

Ordinal data are classified into exhaustive, mutually exclusive, and ordered categories. Ordinal variables allow us to rank the items we measure in terms of which have less and which have more of the quality represented by the variable, but still they do not allow us to say "how *much* more." Using the example of homophobia, if a person were given the statement "I experience homophobia on a daily basis" and asked to respond, the response would fall into one of four categories: "completely agree," "somewhat agree," somewhat disagree," or "completely disagree." The *ordinal measure* consists of those four values. While participants could be rank-ordered between categories, and we would know that a difference exists between categories, we could not say that the differences between categories were necessarily equal.

Interval measurement is based on a unit or interval that permits these units to be measured exactly. Interval scales not only rank-order the items that are measured, but they also quantify and compare the degree of difference between them. Psychological diagnostic tests such as IQ or personality tests are examples of interval measurement.

A *ratio scale* is an interval scale in which distances are stated with respect to a rational zero. Measurement of time, such as the amount of time since your last HIV test, would be an example of a ratio measurement.

Validity

Construct validity refers to how accurately a measure actually reflects the "true" measure of something—in other words, are you measuring what you actually think you are measuring? For example, one might examine whether measures of sexual orientation are actually measuring orientation as theoretically conceived or whether the measure actually captures something else. If the measure had response options that included items related to gender, it might not be considered a valid measure of sexual orientation given that gender is an entirely different construct.

Examples of valid measures can be found when looking at the concept of sexual stigma or internalized homophobia among men and women who identify as gay, lesbian, or bisexual. Among LGB individuals, internalized homophobia refers to the personal acceptance and endorsement of sexual stigma as part of the individual's value system and self-concept (Herek, Gillis, and Cogan 2009). One commonly used measure of internalized homophobia found to have acceptable internal consistency and correlates is the nine-item IHP scale, adapted for self-administration by Herek and Glunt (1995).

Six different indicators can be used to examine the construct validity of a measure:

Face Validity: The content of the measure appears to reflect the construct being measured.
Example: The IHP includes items like "I wish I weren't gay/bisexual" or "I feel alienated from myself because of being gay/bisexual," providing evidence of being face-valid.

Predictive Validity: Scores on the measure predict behaviors on a criterion measured at a future time.
Example: If the measure of internalized homophobia predicted future internalized homophobia, then it would have evidence of predictive validity.

Convergent Validity: Scores on the measure are related to other measures of the same construct.
Example: If scores from the IHP collected at the same time as other measures of internalized homophobia were related to scores from those other measures, then it could be said to have evidence of convergent validity.

Content Validity: The content of the measure is linked to the content that defines the construct.

Example: Internalized homophobia is related to an individual's value system and self-concept. The IHP is content-valid in that it includes items from each of these domains.

Concurrent Validity: Scores on the measures are related to a criterion measured at the same time.
Example: Men scored significantly higher than women on the IHP measure, and bisexuals scored significantly higher than homosexuals, providing evidence of concurrent validity.

Discriminant Validity: Scores on the measure are not related to other measures that are theoretically different.
Example: If the IHP were unrelated to other measures of internalized homophobia, it would indicate that what was being measured was not internalized homophobia and therefore could be said to have evidence of discriminant validity.

Reliability

Reliability refers to the consistency or stability of a measure of behavior. For example, a reliable measure of a psychological variable such as depression will yield the same result each time you administer the depression test to the same person. Any measure that you create comprises two elements: (1) a true score, which is the real score on the variable, and (2) the measurement error. An unreliable measure of depression contains considerable measurement error and therefore does not provide an accurate indication of an individual's true depression. Alternatively, a reliable measure of depression would provide a nearly identical depression score each time the same individual is measured.

Researchers should not use unreliable measures to systematically study variables or the relationships among variables because the results will be unstable and unable to be replicated. In many cases reliability can be increased by making multiples measures: as the number of items increases, so does the reliability. For example, a depression index could have ten or more individual items designed to assess the construct of depression rather than a single measure asking yes/no "are you depressed?"

There are several different methods that one can use to assess reliability. *Test-retest reliability* is assessed by measuring the same individuals at two differing time points. Using two scores for the same person, a correlation coefficient can be calculated, with a higher correlation coefficient being reflective of a higher reliability. While there is no absolute threshold for what a correlation coefficient should be, to consider a measure relatively reliable, it should probably be 0.8 or above. *Internal consistency reliability* is the assessment of reliability using responses from a single time point. If all items are in fact truly measuring the same variable, they should yield consistent results. One indicator of internal consistency reliability is called Cronbach's alpha. The value of the Cronbach's alpha is based on the average of all the inter-item correlation coefficients and the number of items in the measure. A Cronbach's alpha above 0.7 is considered acceptable.

Threats to Quality
Response Biases

Response bias occurs when a group of factors leads a respondent to answer a question incorrectly. Reasons for this include participants' lack of knowledge related to the question or individuals deliberately not wanting to answer the question correctly. The latter may be particularly relevant when surveying LGBTQ populations given sensitivities associated with being a member of this group. The concept of desirability bias (i.e., responses motivated by what is perceived as the socially accepted answer rather than the most accurate one) should be considered by researchers conducting research with LGBTQ individuals. Given that LGBTQ status in and of itself is often considered socially undesirable, research subjects may be additionally primed from the beginning to answer questions differently than their heterosexual counterparts depending on the focus of the study. Response bias ultimately can result in data that are skewed toward a particular way of thinking or behaving that is based on inaccurate information.

In addition to response biases that occur related to particular items or particular study populations, the order in which questions are asked may bias answers. For example, if a survey instrument is particularly long, there is an increased likelihood that attrition will increase toward the end of the survey. In this case, it may be beneficial to randomize the question order to minimize drop off. Furthermore, if particular questions are highly sensitive (e.g. sexual behaviors, substance use, etc.), placing these items toward the middle or end of the survey will allow participants to have had some exposure answering more benign questions and increase their comfort level.

Test Biases

Measurement error relates to the processes involved in data collection. These processes include survey design, format, and wording. Questions that are ambiguous or double-barreled (i.e., asking two different things in a single question) can result in participants selecting an incorrect response option. These types of issues highlight the importance of including response options such as "I don't know" and "I prefer not to answer." In addition to the look and feel of the instrument, the method of data collection can also affect the quality of the data. For example, research has demonstrated that in-person interviews may generate less truthful reporting on sensitive topics than methods that allow respondents to answer the same questions anonymously through, for example, an online survey. Similarly, differences have been found when comparing cross-sectional retrospective reporting of behaviors with prospective longitudinal data collection and when comparing self-report with biomarker data among individuals.

Existing Measurement Tools for Use with LGBTQ Individuals

As a general rule of thumb, when possible, it is preferable to select measures that have been previously created by others and demonstrated to be both valid and reliable, ensuring a maximum level of data integrity from the beginning. *But how does one find existing measures and decide which ones to use?* To start, you should conduct an extensive literature review in your particular area of interest based on the concepts identified in your theoretical framework. By reviewing the literature that has been previously published, you should be able to get a sense of the different items previously used to assess your research focus. Exploration of the literature provides an opportunity to fully evaluate all existing measures related to a particular topic among which you can choose to use in your own study.

In some cases, you may find only a single measurement tool that is appropriate for your use; in other instances, there may be several. Once you have identified the tool(s) that you think might be best suited, it is essential to locate the original publication related to the development of that measure and examine the associated psychometrics. The psychometrics will allow you to understand the strength of a particular measure and gauge its overall validity and reliability. Once you have reviewed the psychometric properties of the chosen measure, you must decide whether you can use the measure in its entirety "as is" or whether you will need to adapt it for your own use.

A few examples of existing measures can easily be found through a literature review; these include:

1. The Sense of Community Scale for use with youth and young adults (Peterson, Speer, and McMillan 2007). This scale assesses sense of community in the LGBTQ community with respect to needs fulfillment, group membership, influence, and emotional connection.
2. The Barriers to Care Scale (BACS), which can be used to measure barriers to health care and other services for LGBTQ people (Heckman et al. 1998). It includes a subscale regarding human service need.
3. A three-item social support scale (e.g., of the people you can talk to and depend on for help, how many of them identify as LGBTQ?) (Wright and Perry, 2006).

In addition to individual items and scales published across journal articles, several books specifically index a variety of different measures to address a wide range of concepts. It is completely appropriate and acceptable to identify these books and use the measures found within.

Adaptation of Existing Measures

You may often find existing measures that are valid but require modification for various reasons. The need to adapt a measure may be related, among other things, to its use with a new population, changes in language that have occurred since the creation of the original measure such as the development of new technology, or the desire to explore new concepts not previously included. Regardless of the reasoning for wanting or needing to adapt an existing measure, it should be understood that these modifications result in measures that require that necessary steps be taken to establish validity.

One example of measure adaptation was conducted by Logie and colleagues, who examined experiences of sexual stigma among LBQ women (Logie and Earnshaw 2015). A previously developed and validated measure titled "The Homophobia Scale" had been used to assess both enacted and perceived/felt-normative stigma based on sexual orientation, racism, and poverty among MSM. While the scale had been used and validated in several subpopulations of MSM (e.g. Black and Latino MSM, MSM living with HIV, and MSM in China), no valid adaptation of the measure was available for use among lesbian, bisexual, or queer-identifying women. The researchers implemented a three-phase validation process beginning with focus groups among the target population to modify the survey items, followed by an internet-based, cross-sectional survey with LBQ women, and a subsequent internet-based survey at two time points with a different group of LBQ women. On completion of data collection, the researchers conducted an exploratory factor analysis yielding one scale with two factors that demonstrated good psychometric properties within the target population.

Creation of New Measures

While the use (or adaptation) of existing measures that have previously been found to be valid and reliable is ideal, in certain circumstances it may be necessary to create entirely new items. Validity in quantitative research can be enhanced by first using qualitative approaches to explore concepts and to identify hypotheses. Qualitative work provides a mechanism to ascertain whether there may be unexplored areas of the topic being studied that *could* yield new items or new contexts for questions (Rowan and Wulff 2007).

In these cases, it should be emphasized that there is a set of best practices for the development of new measures that use qualitative methods to inform the development of quantitative measures. Although a full synopsis of these qualitative approaches is beyond the scope of this chapter, the stages for qualitative work as it relates to item development can be outlined as follows:

Stage 1: Identify Research Questions
Regardless of the approach (i.e., qualitative or quantitative), it is essential to develop a clear set of research questions. The development of research questions should be theoretically rooted and based on your review of the existing scientific literature related to the topic.

Stage 2: Develop Instrument
Given that qualitative data are exploratory in nature, your study instrument will not be a survey but instead will be a guide that helps to facilitate discussion during the data-collection phase. There are different formats of interview and focus group guides, including open-ended, semistructured, and structured. It is important during this stage to create an instrument that captures the domains and concepts you are interested in exploring based on the research questions you developed in Stage 1.

Stage 3: Collect Data
Qualitative research encompasses multiple data-collection methods; most commonly used are individual interviews or focus groups. Similar to the concept of a sample-size calculation in quantitative data collection, qualitative approaches rely on "theoretical saturation" to determine how much data to collect. In short, data should be collected until no new themes or concepts appear to be emerging from new participants and hence the data are saturated.

Stage 4: Analyze Data

Coding describes the process of analyzing qualitative data. Utilizing a grounded-theory approach, coding typically begins with open coding, where an initial constant comparative analysis occurs prior to naming the codes and placing them into categories (Glaser 1992). The data will yield a set of codes that can be subsequently used for the purposes of developing quantitative survey items.

Stage 5: Create Quantitative Survey Items

Based on the data analysis in Stage 4, individual survey items can now be developed and tested. At this stage, the items are still not considered valid or reliable. Survey items should go through the process of pilot testing before being widely disseminated.

Stage 6: Scale Development

Using the results and analysis from the individual items in the survey conducted in Stage 5, it is possible to now assemble items into scale format and go through the process of assessing the psychometric properties of the scale in its entirety.

A more detailed example of this framework, including methodologies such as the use of key informant interviews and analytical approaches (for example, thematic coding), can be found in numerous specialized references, including *Research Design: Qualitative and Quantitative Approaches* (Creswell 2009); *Introduction to Social Research: Quantitative and Qualitative Approaches* (Johnson and Morgan 2016); and *Survey Scales: A Guide to Development, Analysis, and Reporting* (Punch 1998).

Best Practice Considerations

Evolving Social Context Impacting LGBTQ Behaviors, Attitudes, and Norms

While measures themselves are concrete and static, the concepts and constructs that they are used to assess have varying degrees of fluidity. While researchers are trained to be mindful of individual variability when measuring behaviors, attitudes, and norms, increased caution should be applied when doing so among LGBTQ individuals. The ever-evolving social context in which LGBTQ people construct their lives often has a significant impact on the manner in which elements of their lives are measured. As political dynamics, social viewpoints, and public policies shift, so must our ability to revisit and revise measurement tools accordingly. For example, studies examining the impact of relationship status on health outcomes prior to the US Supreme Court's 2015 ruling in *Obergefell v. Hodges* would have used measures that were developed without same-sex marriage being a legal relationship option. Another present-day example of this phenomenon can be seen when examining the healthcare system's use of quality measures for purposes of value-based payment. Quality measures that use sex-specific criteria may inappropriately include or exclude transgender individuals. More large-scale studies must be conducted to incorporate transgender individuals into measures that use sex-specific criteria, and "measure stewards" should consider existing clinical guidelines and recommendations regarding transgender individuals when developing measures. Systems designed exclusively for cisgender individuals will exacerbate transgender healthcare disparities unless they are sufficiently flexible to satisfy transgender individuals' needs.

Measurement of Subpopulations within LGBTQ Communities

As noted throughout this book, LGBTQ individuals represent a distinctive population with unique issues that differ from those of their cisgender heterosexual counterparts. Given the widespread prevalence of disparities among sexual and gender minority individuals, there is a clear need to conduct research that focuses exclusively on LGBTQ persons. However, when conducting such research, it is also critical that researchers and scholars not treat those that fall under the LGBTQ umbrella as a homogenous group, but rather strive to apply and develop measures that are appropriately tailored to subpopulations within varying LGBTQ communities.

LGBTQ individuals who also identify as a person of color are one such understudied subpopulation. A recent study reviewing all research published on Medline during a twenty-year period found that 3,777 articles articles dedicated to public health addressed LGBTQ issues; of these, 85% omitted information on the race/ethnicity of participants (Boehmer 2002). Furthermore, scholarship on minority populations increasingly involves discussion of the significance of understanding the intersections of oppressing identities (Bowleg 2008; Meyer 2010; Stirrat, Meyer, Ouellette, and Gara 2008). However, "while existing measures assess either racism or heterosexism separately for LGBT people of color, there is no existing measure that captures the unique ways that these types of oppressions may intersect for this population." (Balsam, Molina, Beadnell, Simoni, and Walters 2011). For example, although all people of color may experience racism, LGBTQ people of color may be faced with the unique challenge of racist experiences within LGBTQ communities. This raises the possibility that standardized measures of key concepts (e.g., stigma, internalized homophobia) may not be valid and therefore applicable to intersectional populations. These questions represent the next generation of research opportunities in measurement science among LGBTQ populations.

Given the increased visibility and significant burden of disparities faced by individuals identifying as transgender, as well as those who identify as bisexual, an emphasis on both the quantity and quality of research focused exclusively on these populations (which also intersect) is warranted. Prior research has documented a high prevalence of adverse health outcomes in some transgender communities, including mental health distress and suicidality (Clements-Nolle, Marx, Guzman, and Katz 2001; Clements-Nolle, Marx, and Katz 2006; Kenagy 2005), substance use (Hotton, Garofalo, Kuhns, and Johnson 2013), cigarette smoking (Conron, Scott, Stowell, and Landers 2012), and HIV and other STIs (Brennan et al. 2012; Garofalo, Deleon, Osmer, Doll, and Harper 2006; Herbst et al. 2008; Stephens, Bernstein, and Philip 2011). Self-reported data among transgender individuals have documented alarmingly high rates of both depression and attempted suicide (62% and 41%, respectively) (James et al. 2016). Similarly, the percentage of transgender people who have received a new HIV diagnosis is more than three times the national average, with one in four trans women living with HIV (Baral et al. 2013). There also exists a concurrent lack of knowledge, comfort, and skills among health and social service providers who work with transgender clients and patients (Bauer et al. 2009; Hussey 2006; Grossman and D'Augelli 2006; Shires and Jaffee 2015). The combination of biological, psychological, and social factors associated with being a transgender person highlights the complexity of data collection within this subpopulation and the need to create and apply nuanced and culturally appropriate measures. (Hughes, Berzin, Leung, Hersey, and Grallert 2017). Similarly, though bisexual individuals constitute the largest proportion of the "lesbian, gay, and bisexual (LGB)" population, comparatively little research has focused on their unique health concerns and needs. The dearth of research on bisexual health is even more concerning given that bisexual individuals consistently report higher rates of a wide range of negative health outcomes (including mood and anxiety disorders, substance use, suicidality, as well as disparities related to poverty and healthcare access and utilization) when compared with heterosexual and gay/lesbian populations. It is necessary to determine how and why bisexual populations consistently demonstrate disproportionate rates of negative health outcomes relative to their exclusively heterosexual and gay/lesbian counterparts, and also to explore the potential role of resiliency and other factors that may buffer against poor health outcomes among some bisexual individuals.

Conclusions

Our ability to move the field of LGBTQ health forward is heavily dependent on the existence of good measurement. The above discussion represents the foundation and basic principles of scientific measurement through which best practices can be created to ensure we accurately measure health disparities and document them appropriately. As the field of LGBTQ health research continues to advance, it will remain imperative that academics and researchers continue to develop measures specific to new theoretical constructs and newly emerging populations. The tension between new theory and shifting population foci will mean that the subfield of measurement among LGBTQ individuals is contin-

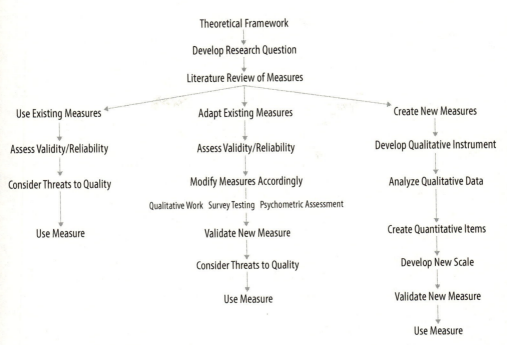

Figure 7.1. Measures decision diagram

uously evolving. While this progression creates a degree of uncertainty, attention to basic measurement approaches (i.e., existing measures, modified measures, new measures) will remain central to facilitating decision-making processes associated with appropriate measurement selection. This chapter provides a brief outline of some of these basic principles and will hopefully prove useful not only in helping individual researchers, but also in facilitating the advancement of empirically driven LGBTQ measurement science. Choosing the "best" measure is an impossible task, as there is not, nor ever will be, any one measure that is universally superior in all contexts. Rather, the goal of this chapter is to emphasize the utility of understanding *how* to make measurement decisions that are evidence based, valid, and reliable.

References

Balsam, K. F., Molina, Y., Beadnell, B., Simoni, J., and Walters, K. 2011. Measuring multiple minority stress: The LGBT People of Color Microaggressions Scale. *Cultural Diversity and Ethnic Minority Psychology* 17: 163–74.

Baral, S. D., Poteat, T., Stromdahl, S., Wirtz, A. L., Guadamuz, T. E., and Beyrer, C. 2013. Worldwide burden of HIV in transgender women: A systematic review and meta-analysis. *Lancet Infectious Diseases* 13: 214–22.

Bauer, G., Hammond, R., Travers, R., Kaay, M., Hohenadel, K., and Boyce, M. 2009. "I don't think this is theoretical; this is our lives": How erasure impacts health care for transgender people. *Journal of the Association of Nurses in AIDS Care* 20: 348–61.

Boehmer, U. 2002. Twenty years of public health research: Inclusion of lesbian, gay, bisexual, and transgender populations. *American Journal of Public Health* 92: 1125–30.

Bowleg, L. 2008. When black + lesbian + woman ≠ black lesbian woman: The methodological challenges of qualitative and quantitative intersectionality research. *Sex Roles* 59: 312–25.

Brennan, J., Kuhns, L. M., Johnson, A. K., Belzer, M., Wilson, E. C., and Garofalo, R. 2012. Syndemic theory and HIV-related risk among young transgender women: The role of multiple, co-occurring health problems and social marginalization. *American Journal of Public Health* 102: 1751–57.

Clements-Nolle, K., Marx, R., Guzman, R., and Katz, M. 2001. HIV prevalence, risk behaviors, health care use, and mental health status of transgender persons: Implications for public health intervention. *American Journal of Public Health* 91: 915–21.

Clements-Nolle, K., Marx, R., and Katz, M. 2006. Attempted suicide among transgender persons: The influence of gender-based discrimination and victimization. *Journal of Homosexuality* 51: 53–69.

Conron, K. J., Scott, G., Stowell, G. S., and Landers, S. J. 2012. Transgender health in Massachusetts: Results from a household probability sample of adults. *American Journal of Public Health* 102: 118–22.

Creswell, J. W. 1994. *Research Design: Qualitative and Quantitative Approaches*. Thousand Oaks, CA: Sage Publications.

Creswell, J. W. 2009. *Research Design: Qualitative, Quantitative, and Mixed-Methods Approaches*. Los Angeles: Sage Publications.

DeVellis, R. F. 2017. *Scale Development: Theory and Applications*. Los Angeles: Sage Publications.

Garofalo, R., Deleon, J., Osmer, E., Doll, M., and Harper, G. W. 2006. Overlooked, misunderstood and at-risk: Exploring the lives and HIV risk of ethnic minority male-to-female transgender youth. *Journal of Adolescent Health* 38: 230–36.

Glaser, B. G. 1992. *Basics of Grounded Theory Analysis*. Mill Valley, CA: Sociology Press.

Grossman, A. H., and D'Augelli, A. R. 2006. Transgender youth: Invisible and vulnerable. *Journal of Homosexuality* 51: 111–28.

Heckman, T., Somlai, A., Peters, J., Walker, J., Otto-Salaj, L., Galdabini, C., and Kelly, J. 1998. Barriers to care among persons living with HIV/AIDS in urban and rural areas. *AIDS Care* 10: 365–375.

Herbst, J. H., Jacobs, E. D., Finlayson, T. J., McKleroy, V. S., Neumann, M. S., and Crepaz, N. 2008. Estimating HIV prevalence and risk behaviors of transgender persons in the United States: A systematic review. *AIDS and Behavior* 12: 1–17.

Herek, G. M., and Glunt, E. K. 1995. Identity and community among gay and bisexual men in the AIDS era: Preliminary findings from the Sacramento Men's Health Study. In G. M. Herek and B. Greene, eds., *AIDS, Identity, and Community: The HIV Epidemic and Lesbians and Gay Men*, 55–84. Thousand Oaks, CA: Sage Publications.

Herek, G. M., Gillis, J. R., and Cogan, J. C. 2009. Internalized stigma among sexual minority adults: Insights from a social psychological perspective. *Journal of Counseling Psychology* 56: 32–43.

Hotton, A. L., Garofalo, R., Kuhns, L. M., and Johnson, A. K. 2013. Substance Use as a Mediator of the Relationship Between Life Stress and Sexual Risk Among Young Transgender Women. *AIDS Education and Prevention* 25: 62–71.

Hughes, L. D., Berzin O. K. G., Leung M., Hersey, C., and Grallert, S. 2017. Adapting healthcare quality measures to transgender individuals. *LGBT Health*, 4, 248–251.

Human Rights Campaign. 2018. *Corporate Equality Index 2018: Rating Workplaces on Lesbian, Gay, Bisexual, Transgender, and Queer Equality*. Available at: https://assets2.hrc.org/files/assets/resources/CEI-2018-FullReport.pdf

Hussey, W. 2006. Slivers of the journey: The use of photovoice and storytelling to examine female to male transsexuals' experience of health care access. *Journal of Homosexuality* 51: 129–58.

Institute of Medicine. 2011. *The Health of Lesbian, Gay, Bisexual, and Transgender People: Building a Foundation for Better Understanding*. Washington, DC: National Academies Press.

James, S. E., Herman, J. L., Rankin, S., Keisling, M., Mottet, L., and Anafi, M. 2016. *The Report of the 2015 U.S. Transgender Survey*. Washington, DC: National Center for Transgender Equality.

Johnson, R. L., and Morgan, G. B. 2016. *Survey Scales: A Guide to Development, Analysis, and Reporting*. New York: Guilford Press.

Kenagy, G. P. 2005. Transgender health: Findings from two needs assessment studies in Philadelphia. *Health Social Work* 30: 19–26.

Logie, C. H., and Earnshaw, V. 2015. Adapting and validating a scale to measure sexual stigma among lesbian, bisexual and queer women. *PLoS ONE* 10: e0116198.

Meyer, I. L. 2010. Identity, stress, and resilience in lesbians, gay men, and bisexuals of color. *Counseling Psychologist* 38: 442–54.

Peterson, N. A., Speer, P., and McMillan, D. 2007. Validation of a brief sense of community scale: Confirmation of the principal theory of sense of community. *Journal of Community Psychology* 36: 61–73.

Punch, K. 1998. *Introduction to Social Research: Quantitative and Qualitative Approaches*. London: Sage Publications.

Rowan, N., and Wulff, D. 2007. Using qualitative methods to inform scale development. *The Qualitative Report* 12: 450–66.

Shires, D. A., and Jaffee, A. 2015. Factors associated with health care discrimination experiences among a national sample of female-to-male transgender individuals. *Health and Social Work* 40: 134–41.

Stephens, S. C., Bernstein, K. T., and Philip, S. S. 2011. Male to female and female to male transgender persons have different sexual risk behaviors yet similar rates of STDs and HIV. *AIDS and Behavior* 15: 683–86.

Stirrat, M. J., Meyer, I. H., Ouellette, S. C., and Gara, M. A. 2008. Measuring identity multiplicity and intersectionality: Hierarchical class analysis (HICLAS) of sexual, racial, and gender identities. *Self and Identity* 7: 89–111.

Strauss, A., and Corbin, J. 1994. Grounded theory methodology: An overview. In N. K. Denzin and Y. S. Lincoln, eds., *Handbook of Qualitative Research*, 273–85. Thousand Oaks, CA: Sage Publications.

Wright, E., and Perry. B. 2006. Sexual identity distress, social support, and the health of gay, lesbian and bisexual youth. *Journal of Homosexuality* 51: 81–110.

EIGHT

Multilevel Approaches to Understanding LGBTQ Health Disparities

Mark L. Hatzenbuehler

WE CANNOT fully understand the determinants of LGBTQ health disparities—and therefore the appropriate level(s) of intervention to reduce these disparities—without considering each level of organization, including individual, dyadic, network, community, and structural. While it is usually not feasible for any one study to examine all of these levels simultaneously, it is nevertheless important to be aware that multiple systems contribute unique variance in explaining LGBTQ health outcomes.

Of course, which level of analysis you focus on in your study depends in large part on your research question. Thus, in the following sections, we explore examples of research at each level of analysis. Because most research has been conducted at the individual level of analysis, and will therefore be most familiar, we only briefly describe illustrative examples of that work. As an organizational framework, we draw in part on Bronfenbrenner's (1979) ecological theory of development, which describes a multisystemic model that nests individuals within increasingly broad systems. This framework is consistent with the socioecological perspective espoused in the 2011 report of the Institute of Medicine on the health of LGBTQ people.

Individual-Level Factors

Factors at the individual level include biopsychosocial factors that affect the health of LGBTQ individuals. Myriad individual-level factors have been examined in the literature, and a full review is beyond the scope of this chapter. Instead, we discuss a few examples to illustrate the range of individual-level factors that have been explored. We divide this section into two classes of risk/protective factors that have been examined at the individual level: factors that are specific to LGBTQ individuals and general psychosocial factors that are common to all individuals, irrespective of their gender identity and sexual orientation.

LGBTQ-Specific Factors

Accumulating evidence indicates that the chronic stress experienced by LGBTQ individuals can be accounted for by experiences that are unique to sexual and gender minorities, including concealment, perceived stigma, and internalized homophobia/transphobia (Meyer 2003a). In addition, a variety of other characteristics and experiences unique to LGBTQ individuals increases the likelihood of exposure to chronic minority stress, including a younger age at coming out, negative reactions to disclosures of sexual orientation and gender identity, and gender nonconformity. Variables specific to LGBTQ individuals, such as perceived stigma because of one's sexual orientation or gender identity, may lead LGBTQ individuals to develop avoidance of certain behaviors or activities, to establish negative thought patterns about the self and others, and ultimately to experience psychological distress (Meyer 2003a). Indeed, these various individual-level characteristics and experiences have been linked to numerous risky behaviors and health outcomes among LGBTQ individuals, including alcohol use, internalizing mental health problems, and suicide risk (Mustanski, Birkett, Greene, Hatzenbuehler, and Newcomb 2014).

General Psychosocial Factors

In contrast to LGBTQ-specific factors, a second class of individual-level factors explores general psychosocial processes (including cognitive, affective, and social processes) that are common to all individuals. This research explores the full range of normative psychological processes through which a sexual and gender minority identity influences development and mental health (e.g., Diamond, Savin-Williams, and Dube 1999). For instance, LGB people are prone to developing deficits in emotion-regulation (Hatzenbuehler 2009; Hatzenbuehler, McLaughlin and Nolen-Hoeksema 2008), which is an established risk factor for psychopathology (Nolen-Hoeksema, Wisco, and Lyubormirsky 2008). Furthermore, evidence from a study of young gay and bisexual men suggests that young people naturally establish resiliency by investing their self-worth in certain domains over which they have more perceived control, such as academic achievement, personal appearance, and competition (Pachankis and Hatzenbuehler 2013). However, overinvestment in these same domains is associated with certain costs, including social isolation, problematic eating, and emotional distress. Thus, it appears that general psychosocial processes risk factors (e.g., emotion regulation, contingencies of self-worth) are often elevated (or suppressed, in the case of protective factors) among LGBTQ individuals, due in part to exposure to stigma-related stressors (Hatzenbuehler 2009).

Structural-Level Factors

In this section, I explore structural-level risk factors for adverse health outcomes among LGBTQ populations. I focus on a particular structural risk factor called *structural stigma*, which refers to "societal-level conditions, cultural norms, and institutional policies and practices that constrain the opportunities, resources, and wellbeing of the stigmatized" (Hatzenbuehler and Link 2014, p. 1). In the first section, I discuss how I became interested in examining structural stigma and review some of the preliminary results that convinced me of the importance of studying this construct. Next, I describe a specific study on structural stigma and LGB health in order to provide an example of how I have approached this research. Finally, I reflect on some of the lessons I have learned in conducting this research, including the challenges and exciting opportunities I see in exploring this line of work.

Why Are Structural Factors Important to LGBTQ Health?

Although theories on determinants of LGB health and sexual orientation-based health disparities have acknowledged the existence as well as the importance of structural factors (Herek 2000; Meyer 2003b), the vast majority of empirical research has been conducted at the individual and interpersonal levels of analysis. This is due in large part to the fact that, until recently, there was little to no variation in structural factors. For instance, the Defense of Marriage Act, passed in 1996, was a federal law that defined marriage as a union that existed only between a man and a woman. Because this institutional form of discrimination affected LGBTQ populations in all 50 states, there was no variability to study—a concept known as a "ubiquitous exposure" (Meyer 2003b). However, once states began to implement their own policies around same-sex marriage and other forms of citizenship rights (e.g., employment nondiscrimination statutes and anti-bullying policies that were inclusive of sexual orientation), there was sufficient variation (and therefore statistical power) to detect an effect, should one exist. This shift in the policy climate coincided with several national, population-based health datasets that started to measure sexual orientation. Thus, datasets finally had all three ingredients that permitted the examination of structural-level factors in shaping LGBTQ health: (1) measures of sexual orientation (and, much less commonly, gender identity); (2) measures of health; and (3) geographic information (e.g., zip code or FIPS code) that enabled researchers to link structural variables (e.g., state-level policies) to individual-level outcomes.

I took advantage of this historic opportunity in one of my dissertation papers. In this study, we coded states for the presence of policies that confer protection to gays and lesbians—namely, hate crime statutes and employment nondiscrimination policies that include sexual orientation as a protected class. We linked this state policy information to individual-level data on mental health and sexual orientation from a nationally representative survey of US adults called the NESARC (National Epidemiologic Survey on Alcohol and Related Conditions). We found that the prevalence of psychiatric disorders was significantly higher among LGB adults living in states with policies that did not confer protection to gays and lesbians, compared with LGB individuals living in states with protective policies (Hatzenbuehler, Keyes, and Hasin 2009). For example, sexual orientation disparities in dysthymia (a mood disorder) were eliminated in states with protective policies; however, LGB adults who lived in states with no protective policies were nearly 2.5 times more likely to meet criteria for dysthymia than were heterosexuals in those same states. These results remained robust after controlling for demographic covariates, as well as for perceived discrimination, suggesting that structural stigma contributes to psychiatric disorders over and above stigma at the individual level.

Knowing This, What Approach Did I Use to Study Structural Stigma in My Next Study?

This study provided some of the very first evidence that structural forms of stigma were associated with adverse mental health outcomes among LGB populations. However, these data were cross-sectional, which is one of the weakest designs for establishing causal inferences. For instance, states with high levels of structural stigma may differ from low-structural stigma states in other ways (e.g., level of income inequality) that are also known to influence health. Although we were able to control for many factors, there is nevertheless the possibility that some third, unmeasured variable is responsible for the results (a process known as unmeasured confounding). I therefore decided that I needed to test the relationship between structural stigma and health using different methodological approaches that would enable us to make stronger causal inferences. Using multiple approaches also affords the opportunity to establish triangulation or convergence across methods, which is another strategy that strengthens causal inference.

One such design is a quasi- or natural experiment (Shadish, Cook, and Campbell 2002). Quasi-experimental studies on structural stigma take advantage of naturally occurring changes, typically changes in social policies (e.g., constitutional amendments banning same-sex marriage). These types of experiments require baseline data before the policy was enacted. Researchers then follow the sample over time to determine any changes in health following the changes in structural stigma.

Although such studies are rare, we identified an opportunity to conduct one such natural experiment. During 2004, numerous states passed constitutional amendments banning same-sex marriage. It so happened that these events occurred between the two waves of data collection in the NESARC (the dataset we used in the study mentioned above). Respondents were first interviewed in 2001 and then the same respondents were re-interviewed in 2005, following the passage of the same-sex marriage bans. This therefore provided a natural experiment that enabled us to examine changes in the prevalence of psychiatric disorders among LGB respondents who were assessed before and after the bans were passed (and also among a heterosexual comparison group).

Results indicated that LGB adults who lived in states that passed same-sex marriage bans experienced a 37% increase in mood disorders, a 42% increase in alcohol use disorders, and a 248% increase in generalized anxiety disorders between the two waves (Hatzenbuehler McLaughlin, Keyes, and Hasin 2010). In contrast, LGB adults living in states without these bans did not experience a statistically significant increase in psychiatric disorders during the study period. Moreover, the mental health of heterosexuals in states that passed the bans was largely unchanged during this period, which provided further evidence for result specificity and gave us greater confidence that these relationships were causal.

What Did We Learn from This Approach?

In these two studies—and in several follow-up studies that have used different designs and measures of structural stigma (for a review, see Hatzenbuehler 2014)—we found that structural stigma has wide-ranging impacts for the health of sexual minorities, ranging from mal-adaptive physiological stress responses in the laboratory (Hatzenbuehler and McLaughlin 2014) to premature mortality at a population level (Hatzenbuehler, Bellatorre, Lee, Finch, Muennig, and Fiscella 2014).

Although this work has opened up new avenues for understanding structural determinants of LGBTQ health, as well as for identifying policy-level interventions to reduce these disparities, it is not without its challenges (similar to the other levels of analysis explored in this chapter). One challenge involves measurement. Existing measures of stigma were largely developed to ask respondents about their percep-tions of stigma and their experiences of interpersonal discrimination, rather than to investigate structural forms of stigma (Meyer 2003b). Consequently, studying structural stigma requires the development of new measures capable of reliably capturing this construct. Another chal-lenge involves data structures. As previously mentioned, to evaluate the health consequences of structural stigma, researchers require large-scale studies occurring over multiple geographic regions—neighborhoods, counties, or states—that offer sufficient variation in levels of structural stigma in order to detect an effect. It is often difficult to find such data-sets, especially because of the lack of population-based datasets with measures of sexual orientation and gender identity, which is itself a marker of structural stigma. However, this is increasingly changing, as several datasets, including the national Youth Risk Behavior Surveil-lance study and the National Health Interview Survey, have begun to add measures of sexual orientation to their surveys.

Despite these challenges, there are many rewarding aspects of this work. One in particular has been that several of our studies have been cited in *amicus curiae* (friend of the court) briefs for court cases on sex-ual orientation-based discrimination. This work therefore provides a compelling example of the use of social science data in court cases that seek to eliminate discrimination against LGBTQ individuals.

There are also several exciting directions for expanding this research on structural stigma and LGBTQ health. First, as this work is still in its relative infancy, the next generation of research will benefit from identifying mediators and moderators of the structural stigma-health association. That is, why does structural stigma affect LGBTQ health, and what factors either strengthen or undermine the impact of structural stigma on the health of LGBTQ individuals? Second, the approach that we have used can be adapted to a global context in order to explore how structural-level factors affect LGBTQ individuals in countries that continue to enact discriminatory laws and policies that target LGBTQ populations. Third, only one study has examined structural stigma and the health of transgender populations (Perez-Brumer, Hatzenbuehler, Oldenberg, Bockting, in press). As in research on LGB populations, there has been very little variation in structural stigma surrounding gender minorities. However, the policy climate around transgender citizenship rights is rapidly changing, permitting the examination of structural forms of stigma that are specific to this group and linking these factors to health outcomes among transgender respondents.

Conclusions

In this chapter, we have reviewed illustrative examples of research on LGBTQ health exploring risk and protective factors across multiple levels of organization, ranging from the individual to the structural. Although we discussed these levels separately, they do not exist in isolation. Indeed, there is likely a dynamic interplay among these levels, which suggests that changes at one level may alter determinants at other levels (Mustanski et al. 2014). It is increasingly possible to empirically test that hypothesis, as studies now routinely collect measures across several levels of analysis (e.g., National Longitudinal Study of Adolescent Health), and methods are available for handling multilevel data (e.g., hierarchical linear modeling). Thus, while it is clear that addressing LGBTQ disparities requires research at each level of analysis, it will be important for future studies to examine cross-level influences in order to obtain a more comprehensive understanding of determinants of LGBTQ health.

Useful References for Students to Read as Possible Assignments
    Hatzenbuehler, M. L. 2011. The social environment and suicide attempts in a population-based sample of LGB youth. *Pediatrics* 127: 896–903.

Hatzenbuehler, M. L., Bellatorre, A., Lee, Y., Finch, B., Muennig, P., and Fiscella, K. 2014. Structural stigma and all-cause mortality in sexual minority populations. *Social Science & Medicine* 103: 33–41.

Hatzenbuehler, M. L., Keyes, K. M., and Hasin, D. S. 2009. State-level policies and psychiatric morbidity in lesbian, gay, and bisexual populations. *American Journal of Public Health* 99: 2275–81.

Hatzenbuehler, M. L., McLaughlin, K. A., Keyes, K. M., and Hasin, D. S. 2010. The impact of institutional discrimination on psychiatric disorders in lesbian, gay, and bisexual populations: A prospective study. *American Journal of Public Health* 100: 452–59.

Hatzenbuehler, M. L., O'Cleirigh, C., Grasso, C., Mayer, K., Safren, S., and Bradford, J. 2012. Effect of same-sex marriage laws on health care use and expenditures in sexual minority men: A quasi-natural experiment. *American Journal of Public Health* 102: 285–91.

References

Bronfenbrenner, U. 1979. *The Ecology of Human Development: Experiments by Nature and Design.* Cambridge, MA: Harvard University Press.

Diamond, L. M., Savin-Williams, R. C., and Dube, E. M. (1999. Sex, dating, passionate friendships and romance: Intimate peer relations among lesbian, gay, and bisexual adolescents. In W. Furman, C. Feiring, and B. B. Brown, eds., *Contemporary Perspectives on Adolescent Romantic Relationships,* 175–210. New York: Cambridge University Press.

Hatzenbuehler, M. L. 2014. Structural stigma and the health of lesbian, gay, and bisexual populations. *Current Directions in Psychological Science* 23(2): 127–32.

Hatzenbuehler, M. L. 2009. How does sexual minority stigma "get under the skin"? A psychological mediation framework. *Psychological Bulletin* 135(5): 707–30.

Hatzenbuehler, M. L., Bellatorre, A., Lee, Y., Finch, B., Muennig, P., and Fiscella, K. 2014. Structural stigma and all-cause mortality in sexual minority populations. *Social Science & Medicine* 103: 33–41.

Hatzenbuehler, M. L., Keyes, K. M., and Hasin, D. S. 2009. State-level policies and psychiatric morbidity in lesbian, gay, and bisexual populations. *American Journal of Public Health* 99(12): 2275–81.

Hatzenbuehler, M. L., and Link, B. G. 2014. Introduction to the special issue on structural stigma and health. *Social Science & Medicine* 103: 1–6.

Hatzenbuehler, M. L., and McLaughlin, K. A. 2014. Structural stigma and hypothalamic-pituitary-adrenocortical axis reactivity in lesbian, gay, and bisexual young adults. *Annals of Behavioral Medicine* 47(1): 39–47.

Hatzenbuehler, M. L., McLaughlin, K. A., and Nolen-Hoeksema, S. 2008. Emotion regulation and internalizing symptoms in a longitudinal study of sexual minority and heterosexual adolescents. *Journal of Child Psychology and Psychiatry* 49(12): 1270–78.

Hatzenbuehler, M. L., McLaughlin, K. A., Keyes, K. M., and Hasin, D. S. 2010. The impact of institutional discrimination on psychiatric disorders in lesbian, gay, and bisexual populations: A prospective study. *American Journal of Public Health* 100(3): 452–59.

Herek, G. M. 2000. The psychology of sexual prejudice. *Current Directions in Psychological Science* 9(1): 19–22.

Institute of Medicine. 2011. Committee on Lesbian Gay Bisexual and Transgender Health Issues and Research Gaps and Opportunities. *The Health of Lesbian, Gay, Bisexual, and Transgender People: Building a Foundation for Better Understanding.* Washington, DC: National Academies Press.

Meyer, I. H. 2003a. Prejudice, social stress, and mental health in lesbian, gay, and bisexual populations: Conceptual issues and research evidence. *Psychological Bulletin* 129(5): 674–97.

Meyer, I. H. 2003b. Prejudice as stress: Conceptual and measurement problems. *American Journal of Public Health* 93(2): 262–65.

Mustanski, B., Birkett, M., Greene, G., Hatzenbuehler, M. L., and Newcomb, M. 2014. Envisioning an America without sexual orientation inequities in adolescent health. *American Journal of Public Health* 104(2): 218–25.

Nolen-Hoeksema, S., Wisco, B. E., and Lyubormirsky, S. 2008. Rethinking rumination. *Perspectives on Psychological Science* 3(5): 400–24.

Pachankis, J. E., and Hatzenbuehler, M. L. 2013. The social development of contingent self-worth in sexual minority young men: An empirical investigation of the *Best Little Boy in the World* hypothesis. *Basic and Applied Social Psychology* 35(2): 176–90.

Perez-Brumer, A., Hatzenbuehler, M. L., Oldenberg, C., and Bockting, W. 2015. Individual- and structural-level risk factors for suicide attempts among transgender individuals. *Behavioral Medicine* 41(3): 164–71

Shadish, W., Cook, T., and Campbell, D. 2002. *Experimental and Quasi-Experimental Designs for Generalized Causal Inference.* Boston: Houghton Mifflin Co.

NINE

Social-Network Approaches to HIV Prevention and Care

Carl Latkin and Karin E. Tobin

WESTERN SOCIETIES that emphasize individualism often ignore or downplay social factors and their role in changing health behaviors. Yet social factors are often more powerful determinants of behavior than individual-level attributes. But how do we understand social factors and use them in developing interventions for promoting health behaviors? A major focus of our research team has been to delineate how the social context influences risk behaviors and how we can capitalize on microsocial structures and naturally occurring social processes to promote health behavior change.[1-4] Moreover, it is important to understand how we can alter social dynamics so that they are sustained by the social environment, institutions, and policies. In developing microsocial influence-oriented interventions, it is critical to ask: who are the important people in the lives of our participants, and how might these relationships influence health behaviors?

Social-network measures are a systematic method to delineate these key individuals. A social network has been defined as individuals linked to a focal individual by a particular behavior or interaction, e.g., support exchange, sexual contact, drug sharing.[5] Network members may include multiple social spheres of influence, such as sex or drug partners, friends, family, neighbors, and coworkers.

Social-network members are main sources of social environmental information that individuals receive for self-monitoring their behaviors. Social network members have been found to have powerful influences on individuals' behaviors, including through processes of norm formation and maintenance, social comparison and social control, and fear of social sanctions. Because of the social nature of HIV transmission, inclusion of social-network factors in prevention efforts is essential.

Social networks have been theorized to comprise structural and relational components.[6] Structures of personal networks have been found to have implications for risk behavior and HIV prevention. Structural characteristics of personal networks include number of sex partners, density and overlap of function, termed multiplexity (e.g., financial support), and sex partner.

Social-network factors have been found to be associated with HIV and STI transmission.[7-9] Indeed, there is evidence that network structural characteristics (e.g., network density and connectivity) and dynamics (e.g., partner concurrency) may lead to high rates of infectious diseases.[10-12] Network dynamics have also been used to explain the greater burden of HIV/AIDS among African Americans compared with other racial groups in the United States, even within communities with similar levels of HIV risk behaviors.[13]

Peers are important sources of influence on sexual and drug use behaviors. Peers may influence each other's risk behaviors through social comparison processes, fear of social sanctions, information exchange, socialization of new group members, modeling and reinforcement, and social interactions that provide opportunities to meet new sex partners.

Personal network structure and relational characteristics are associated with HIV risk behaviors, including having multiple partners and exchanging sex for money or drugs,[14-18] and norms of sexual risk behaviors.[17] Network dynamics have also been used to explain racial differences in HIV rates.[13] Smith et al. reported that among a predominantly White MSM sample, a higher-density network was associated with lower sex risk, and a mixed HIV serostatus network was associated with a higher number of anal sex partners.[19] This finding may be attributable to social monitoring of network members' behaviors or to peer norms that favored safer behavior.

Sexual partner characteristics have been identified as HIV risk factors.[20] We have found that condom use among African American drug-using populations is also associated with financial interdependence, partners' drug use, and a range of measures of intimacy.[21] Age mixing may partially explain HIV seroprevalence patterns and racial differences among young gay men[22] and African American MSM.[20] Among a sample of MSM in Los Angeles who were majority gay-identified, African American MSM were more likely to report having sex with a different-aged sex partner compared with other racial groups, and they were more likely to report having an African American male anal sex partner compared with other racial groups.[20]

In Baltimore, we found social network differences between African American MSM who have sex only with men and those who have sex with men and women.[23] The majority of both groups report kin in their networks, and most report people living with HIV in their social networks. About 40% of the participants reported that their sexual partners provide emotional support. Men who had sex with both men and women reported greater concurrency of sexual partnerships.

In other analyses of social-network characteristics of African American MSM, we found that receiving emotional support from a family member or a sex partner was associated with reduced odds of having depressive symptoms.[24] Disclosure of same-sex behavior to a network member was associated with being HIV positive, the network member being positive, the network member providing emotional support, and not being a female sexual partner.[25] Whereas disclosure of HIV-positive status was associated with a network member lending money to the participant, emotional support, and network members' positive HIV status. Attributes of social network members associated with disclosure of positive serostatus included the network member being older, HIV positive, providing emotional support, lending money, and not being a male sex partner.

Intervention Development

We have developed and tested randomized clinical trials of social network–oriented interventions in a range of minority and stigmatized populations.[26-28] The goal of these interventions has been to promote behavior change not only among those individuals who receive the interventions, but also among their social network members who do not directly receive the intervention. This approach allows for promoting behavior change among individuals who may not want or be able to enroll in an intervention due to lack of resources, concerns about stigmatization and disclosure, perceived relevance, and competing priorities.

In intervention development, the question of the diversity of the target audience often arises. There is a wide range of gender expressions and salience of these expressions among African American MSM. Moreover, there is variation by age, economic and employment status, education, drug use, disclosure of same-sex behavior, HIV status, and the genders of partners. So how do you develop interventions that address this spectrum of participants? If an intervention does not address a sufficiently diverse population, it is unlikely that it will be disseminated, as most health departments and NGOs cannot run numerous interventions.

Another issue in developing social influence interventions is how to facilitate conversations about HIV prevention and medical care so that such conversations become normative. In our research we have found that despite positive attitudes toward talking about HIV topics with peers, most participants reported that they talked to very few social network members about such topics as HIV testing.

In developing interventions, we have endeavored to promote network-level behavior change by fostering self-identities associated with encouraging others to engage in health behaviors. The interventions are also designed to provide social rewards for promoting the new behavior and to establish new social norms that promote discussing health behaviors and risk reduction. Factors that we have focused on in developing network-oriented interventions include:

- Identifying stable sources of influence for health behaviors
- Identifying motives for participants to reduce their own risk behaviors and to promote risk reduction among their social networks
- Providing training in communications skills to promote network risk reduction
- Ensuring that intervention social roles, identities, and materials enhance participants' credibility in the community regarding health promotion
- Providing support and feedback to peer educators through small group sessions
- Including activities at each session that are practiced with their network members in the community
- Evaluating behavior change in the peer educators and their network members while minimizing social desirability response bias.

Our interventions are based on theory, yet these theories do not tell us which intervention components will be effective or even which components are critical to include in an intervention. Moreover, participants' reports of satisfaction with intervention content are not a good measure of the likelihood that the intervention will produce behavior change.

Our network interventions involve active learning, including realistic scenarios, practicing new behaviors, modeling by facilitators, and reviews of experiences outside of the intervention group (homework) in promoting behavior change among network members and others in the community. These intervention activities are designed to increase salience of health-promotion social norms within networks. As social norms within networks are often contradictory, the conversations focus on heightening the norms for promoting health behaviors. These conversations enhance the acceptability and frequency of talking about HIV-related behavior. Through social diffusion processes, behavior change is hypothesized to flow through the social networks.

Another key aspect of social interventions is developing social roles that promote risk reduction and can be sustained. Developing a social identity valued by the community can help accomplish this goal. The social identity and behaviors of promoting risk-reduction behaviors can be sustained by positive feedback from individuals' social networks as well as from the intervention group.

Our initial network intervention for African MSM (Unity in Diversity) was based in part on findings from interventions for other key populations.[29] We anticipated that individuals who adopt a "peer mentor" identity would be motivated to promote and endorse HIV preventive behaviors, and that their advocacy and modeling of safer behaviors will introduce safer sex and drug norms to their network members. Furthermore, it was hypothesized that peer outreach would alter norms about risk reduction and HIV/STI testing within social networks and consequently lead to behavior change. To address the potential heterogeneity of sexual orientation/identity and disclosure of risk behavior, the intervention focused on peer outreach, not sexual identity, as a means to community empowerment.

The Unity in Diversity intervention incorporated a mix of complementary components from Information-Motivation-Behavior Skills Model, Social Cognitive Theory, Social Identity Theory, Social Norms, Cognitive Dissonance, and Diffusion of Innovations Theory[30–33] to target the multifaceted factors that are associated with risk behavior and testing, and address the diversity of needs, motivations, and circumstances of African American MSM. We designed the intervention to provide African American MSM an opportunity to perform a social role of peer health educator that encourages HIV testing and risk reduction without focusing on stigmatizing identities or behaviors. We encouraged participants to promote testing and risk reduction with all of their social network members, male and female. Through discussion of HIV prevention and testing, we expected that social network members will reinforce health promotion behaviors and that peer outreach will facilitate behavior change among the peer health educators. As many participants had been bombarded by messages about HIV, the focus on the intervention was men's sexual health.

The intervention was a seven-session (six group-based and one individual session) randomized clinical trial. To capitalize on social influence processes, the intervention was delivered in small group-based sessions, which enabled participants to learn from their peers' experiences and to establish and promote social norms about condom use and testing. Role-play activities were included so that participants could practice and role-model communication skills. Sessions included numerous opportunities to practice these new skills.

Recruitment occurred at bars, clubs, cafes, restaurants, and college campuses. Print advertisements were placed in local and university-based newspapers. Referrals were obtained from agencies that provide services to African American MSM. We also conducted internet-based recruitment. A total of 147 participants were randomized between the intervention (n=75) and control conditions (n=72). Retention was high, as 96% of participants in the intervention condition (n=73) and control condition (n=71) completed the follow-up assessment.

At the three-month follow-up assessment, we found statistically significant differences between the comparison and experimental groups. Specifically, being in the intervention condition was associated with increased odds of condom use with male partners (adjusted odds ratio, $AOR = 2.64$, 95% $CI = 0.95$–7.36) and HIV-negative/unknown status partners ($AOR = 3.19$, 95% $CI = 0.98$–10.38) at follow-up.

Based on these findings, we have embarked on a larger randomized clinical trial with a greater number of participants and a longer duration for the follow-up assessments. In Unity in Diversity, we found that it was difficult for index participants to recruit their network members prior to experiencing the intervention, perhaps due to a lack of trust and competing priorities. Consequently, we changed the approach so that the indexes recruited network members for HIV testing and counseling after the index participants had received intervention sessions (rather than before) and hence had learned communication skills for promoting risk reduction and HIV testing among their network members. We also found that the role of peer educator did not initially resonate with participants. Hence, the role was modified and framed as taking care of self, friends, and community.

Although social network–oriented interventions for minority urban MSM sound appealing, there are impediments and barriers to behavior change that need to be taken into consideration in developing effective interventions. One key issue is how do you make interventions relevant to participants when they have other priorities? Often among urban racial minority MSM, a high percentage is seeking employment and is experiencing violence in their neighborhoods, police harassment, and high levels of incarceration. Moreover, in communities with a minimal number of organizations that support sexual minority health, there is the pressing issue of how to foster a supportive community for sexual minorities.

There is a need for structural interventions to develop community organizations to promote the physical and mental health of racial minority MSM in impoverished urban areas, train members of the community in leadership roles, and integrate sexual minority health care with other activities. Interventions should also address the high levels of unemployment, violence, and incarceration among these populations. In the realm of research approaches and methods, there is a need for more qualitative analyses of the social dynamics that lead to health promotion conversations and the documentation of successful approaches used by community members to overcome barriers to health promotion. Although our social-network approach to HIV prevention and care among African American MSM is promising, we must not forget the individual, social, and structural factors that foster the epidemic and impede HIV prevention and appropriate medical care for those living with HIV.

References

1. Latkin, C., Yang, C., Tobin,, K., and Hulbert A. 2010. Factors associated with recruiting an HIV seropositive risk network member among injection drug users. *AIDS and Behavior* 14(5): 1137–41.

2. Bohnert, A. S., German, D., Knowlton, A. R., and Latkin, C. A. 2010. Friendship networks of inner-city adults: A latent class analysis and multi-level regression of supporter types and the association of supporter latent class membership with supporter and recipient drug use. *Drug and Alcohol Dependence* 107(2–3): 134–40.

3. Latkin, C. A., Kuramoto, S. J., Davey-Rothwell, M. A., and Tobin, K. E. 2010. Social norms, social networks, and HIV risk behavior among injection drug users. *AIDS and Behavior* 14(5): 1159–68.

4. Costenbader, E. C., Astone, N. M., and Latkin, C. A. 2006. The dynamics of injection drug users' personal networks and HIV risk behaviors. *Addiction* 101(7): 1003–13.

5. Miller, R. L., Klotz, D., and Eckholdt, H. M. 1998. HIV prevention with male prostitutes and patrons of hustler bars: Replication of an HIV preventive intervention. *American Journal of Community Psychology* 26(1): 97–131.

6. Hall, A., and Wellman, B. 1985. Social networks and social support. In S. Cohen and L. Syme, eds., *Social Support and Health*. New York: Academic Press.

7. Friedman, S. R., Neaigus. A., Jose, B., Curtis, R., Goldstein, M., Ildefonso, G., Rothenberg, R. B., and Des Jarlais, D. C. 1997. Sociometric risk networks and risk for HIV infection. *American Journal of Public Health* 87(8): 1289–96.

8. Périssé, A. R., Langenberg, P., Hungerford, L., Boulay, M., Charurat, M., Schechter, M., and Blattner. W. 2010. Egocentric network data provide additional information for characterizing an individual's HIV risk profile. *AIDS* 24(2): 291–98.

9. Ward, H. 2007. Prevention strategies for sexually transmitted infections: Importance of sexual network structure and epidemic phase. *Sexually Transmitted Infections* 83 Suppl 1: i43–i49.

10. Adimora, A. A., Schoenbach, V. J., and Doherty, I. A. 2006. HIV and African Americans in the southern United States: Sexual networks and social context. *Sexually Transmitted Diseases* 33(7 Suppl): S39–S45.

11. Choudhury, B., Risley, C. L., Ghani, A. C., Bishop, C. J., Ward, H., Fenton, K. A., Ison, C. A., and Spratt, B. G. 2006. Identification of individuals with gonorrhea within sexual networks: A population-based study. *Lancet* 368(9530): 139–46.

12. Morris, M., and Kretzschmar, M. 1995. Concurrent partnerships and transmission dynamics in networks. *Social Networks* 17(3–4): 299–318.

13. Kottiri, B. J., Friedman, S. R., Neaigus, A., Curtis, R., and Des Jarlais, D. C. 2002. Risk networks and racial/ethnic differences in the prevalence of HIV infection among injection drug users. *Journal of Acquired Immune Deficiency Syndromes* 30(1): 95–104.

14. DiClemente, R. J., Wingood, G. M., Crosby, R. A., Sionean, C., Cobb, B. K., Harrington, K., Davies, S. L, Hook, E. W., III, and Oh, M. K. 2002. Sexual risk behaviors associated with having older sex partners: A study of black adolescent females. *Sexually Transmitted Diseases* 29(1):20–24.

15. Ford, K., Sohn, W., and Lepkowski, J. 2002. American adolescents: Sexual mixing patterns, bridge partners, and concurrency. *Sexually Transmitted Diseases* 29(1): 13–19.

16. Latkin, C., Mandell, W., Vlahov, D., Oziemkowska, M., and Celentano, D. 1996. People and places: Behavioral settings and personal network characteristics as correlates of needle sharing. *Journal of Acquired Immune Deficiency Syndromes and Human Retrovirology* 13(3): 273–80.

17. Latkin, C. A., Forman, V., Knowlton, A., and Sherman, S. 2003. Norms, social networks, and HIV-related risk behaviors among urban disadvantaged drug users. *Social Science & Medicine* 56(3): 465–76.

18. Miller, M., and Neaigus, A. 2001. Networks, resources and risk among women who use drugs. *Social Science & Medicine* 52(6): 967–78.

19. Smith, A. M., Grierson, J., Wain, D., Pitts, M., and Pattison, P. 2004. Associations between the sexual behaviour of men who have sex with men and the structure and composition of their social networks. *Sexually Transmitted Infections* 80(6): 455–58.

20. Bingham, T. A., Harawa, N. T., Johnson, D. F., Secura, G. M., MacKellar, D. A., and Valleroy, L. A. 2003. The effect of partner characteristics on HIV infection among African American men who have sex with men in the Young Men's Survey, Los Angeles, 1999–2000. *AIDS Education and Prevention* 15(1 Suppl A): 39–52.

21. Sherman, S. G., and Latkin, C. A. 2001. Intimate relationship characteristics associated with condom use among drug users and their sex partners: A multilevel analysis. *Drug and Alcohol Dependency* 64(1): 97–104.

22. Morris, M., Zavisca, J., and Dean, L. 1995. Social and sexual networks: Their role in the spread of HIV/AIDS among young gay men. *AIDS Education and Prevention* 7(5 Suppl): 24–35.

23. Latkin. C. A., Yang, C., Tobin, K., Penniman, T., Patterson, J., and Spikes, P. 2011. Differences in the social networks of African American men who have sex with men only and those who have sex with men and women. *American Journal of Public Health* 101(10): e18–e23.

24. Yang, C., Latkin, C., Tobin, K., Patterson, J., and Spikes, P. 2013. Informal social support and depression among African American men who have sex with men. *Journal of Community Psychology* 41(4): 435–45.

25. Latkin, C., Yang, C., Tobin, K., Roebuck, G., Spikes, P., and Patterson. J. 2012. Social network predictors of disclosure of MSM behavior and HIV-positive serostatus among African American MSM in Baltimore, Maryland. *AIDS and Behavior* 16(3): 535–42.

26. Davey-Rothwell, M. A., Tobin, K., Yang, C., Sun, C. J., and Latkin, C. A. 2011. Results of a randomized controlled trial of a peer mentor HIV/STI prevention intervention for women over an 18 month follow-up. *AIDS and Behavior* 15(8): 1654–63.

27. Latkin, C. A., Donnell, D., Metzger, D., Sherman, S., Aramrattna, A., Davis-Vogel, A., Quan, V. M., Gandham, S., Vongchak, T., Perdue, T., and Celentano, D. D. 2009. The efficacy of a network intervention to reduce HIV risk behaviors among drug users and risk partners in Chiang Mai, Thailand, and Philadelphia, USA. *Social Science & Medicine* 68(4): 740–48.

28. Tobin, K. E., Kuramoto, S. J., Davey-Rothwell, M. A., and Latkin, C. A. 2011. The STEP into Action study: A peer-based, personal risk network–focused HIV prevention intervention with injection drug users in Baltimore, Maryland. *Addiction* 106(2): 366–75.

29. Tobin, K., Kuramoto, S. J., German D., Fields E., Spikes P. S., Patterson J., and Latkin, C. 2013. Unity in diversity: results of a randomized clinical culturally tailored pilot HIV prevention intervention trial in Baltimore, Maryland, for African American men who have sex with men. *Health Education and Behavior* 40(3): 286–95.

30. Rogers, E. 2003. *Diffusion of Innovations.* 5th ed. New York: Free Press.

31. Fisher, J. D., Fisher, W. A., Amico, K. R., and Harman J. J. 2006. An information-motivation-behavioral skills model of adherence to antiretroviral therapy. *Health Psychology* 25(4): 462–73.

32. Turner, J. C. 1978. Social comparison and social identity: Some perspectives for intergroup behavior. *European Journal of Social Psychology* 5:5–34.

33. Bandura, A. 1986. *Social Foundations of Thought and Action: A Social Cognitive Theory.* Englewood Cliffs, NJ: Prentice-Hall.

[TEN]

Why Focus on Gay Couples in HIV Prevention Research?

Colleen Hoff

HIV INFECTION rates among gay men remain high, and for those who are in relationships infection is increasingly attributed to primary partners. Research shows that between 40% and 68% of HIV infections among gay men in the United States are the result of unprotected sex with infected primary partners (Davidovich et al. 2001; Goodreau et al. 2012; Sullivan, Salazar, Buchbinder, and Sanchez 2009). These data are the most recent to confirm a trend already noted in past research. That is, men in relationships engage in substantially higher rates of unprotected anal intercourse with their primary partner as compared with single men with nonprimary partners (Bosga et al. 1995; Cáceres and Rosasco 1997; Connell et al. 1990; Ekstrand, Stall, Paul, Osmond, and Coates 1999; Elford, Bolding, Maguire, and Sherr 1999; Fitzpatrick, McLean, Dawson, Boulton, and Hart 1990; Hays, Kegeles, and Coates, 1990; Hays, Kegeles, and Coates 1997; Hoff, Coates, Barrett, Collette, and Ekstrand 1996; Hoff et al. 1997; Hope and MacArthur 1998; Kippax, Crawford, Davis, Rodden, and Dowsett 1993; Martin, Dean, Garcia, and Hall 1989; McKusick, Coates, Morin, Pollack, and Hoff 1990; Schmidt et al. 1992; Stall, Ekstrand, Pollack, McKusick, and Coates 1990; Valdiserri et al. 1988). Further, men in relationships who share the same serostatus report higher rates of condomless sex than men who do not share the same serostatus (Hoff 1998; Hoff et al. 1997; Hoff and SUMS Team 1999; Kippax et al. 1997; Stall, Hays, Waldo, Ekstrand, and McFarland 2000). However, little is known about why more risk behavior is occurring among men in relationships, and specifically, what dynamics within a relationship may contribute to this phenomenon. Given that approximately 50% of gay men are in primary relationships (Adib, Joseph, Ostrow, Tal, and Schwartz 1991; Blumstein and Schwartz 1983; Bosga et al. 1995; Cáceres and Rosasco 1997; Choi, Coates, Catania, Lew, and Chow 1995; Díaz, Morales, Bein, Dilán, and Rodríguez 1999; Halkitis, Wilton, Parsons, and Hoff 2004; Harry 1984; Hoff et al. 1996; Hoff et al. 1997; Kegeles, Hays, and Coates 1996; Kippax et al. 1993; McKusick et al. 1990; Peplau, Cochran, and Mays 1997; Saghir and Robins 1973), it is vital to gain a better understanding of this group largely overlooked in HIV prevention.

Background Literature

There are a limited number of studies of HIV prevention interventions targeting gay couples. The limited number of couples interventions is not surprising given that the behavior change models commonly used in HIV prevention are individually focused models (Becker 1974; Fishbein and Ajzen 1975; Janz and Becker 1984). For example, the AIDS Risk Reduction Model (ARRM) states that individuals must (a) label their behaviors as problematic, (b) make a personal commitment to change risky behaviors, and (c) enact the changes. According to this model, labeling behaviors as problematic is dependent upon perception of susceptibility to HIV infection, in addition to knowledge of which sexual activities are associated with HIV transmission and a belief that AIDS is life-threatening. Without labeling the behaviors as risky and believing that one is personally susceptible, change is unlikely to occur (Catania, Kegeles, and Coates 1990). This and other models of behavior change are helpful, but they leave out the important interpersonal dynamics at play between partners.

Interdependence-based models provide a helpful foundation from which to build theories of risk reduction for couples. In general, interdependence theory focuses on the interaction between partners in close relationships (Drigotas, Rusbult, and Verette 1999; Rempel, Holmes, and Zanna, 1985; Wieselquist, Rusbult, Foster, and Agnew 1999). It is especially concerned with the interdependence between two individuals and each partner's ability to influence the other's behavior. One specific area of interdependence theory that is worthy of further investigation, as it relates to HIV risk behavior, is the process of "transformation of motivation." Interdependence theory posits that within relationships there are ongoing shifts between "given preferences," behavioral preferences based on immediate, self-centered reactions to an event, and "effective preferences," preferences based on the implicit or explicit consideration of long-term consequences, implications for the partner, and broader concerns (e.g., concern for the well-being of the relationship) (Arriaga and Rusbult 1998; Kelley and Thibaut 1978). Thus, the process of transformation of motivation, whereby couples relinquish their immediate self-interests and act in the interest of the relationship (Rusbult and Buunk 1993), is a compelling issue with regard to sexual risk-taking behavior among couples. For example, if an HIV-negative partner avoids bringing up his discomfort about engaging in condomless anal sex with his HIV-positive partner "for the good of the relationship," a meaningful opportunity to intervene with couples is lost.

A prevention strategy introduced by Kippax (1997) and her colleagues known as "negotiated safety" posited that two seronegative partners agree to have only safe sex or no sex outside the relationship in order to have unprotected anal sex within the relationship. Studies addressing the effectiveness of this strategy are mixed. One study reported that couples who had negotiated safety agreements were safer than those who did not have these agreements (Kippax et al. 1993). Another study reported that couples had difficulty adhering to some of the main components of a negotiated safety agreement such as knowing one's HIV status and having unprotected sex with outside partners (Elford et al. 1999).

Building upon the negotiated safety literature, Hoff and Beougher (2010) found that agreements about sex with outside partners are ubiquitous and integral to nearly all gay male couples regardless of couple serostatus. They also found that sexual agreements serve as a framework for the couples' decision to engage in, or refrain from, sexual behaviors that may place them at increased risk for HIV. Given the level of unprotected anal intercourse (UAI) among gay couples, elucidating the role these agreements play in gay men's sexual decision-making and in their relationships is imperative for HIV prevention.

Other relationship factors such as intimacy and emotional closeness are associated with sexual risk-taking (Bosga et al. 1995). Barrier methods of HIV prevention, such as condom use, are quite literally perceived as barriers to intimacy and relationship satisfaction. Research involving diverse samples points to a consistent association between unprotected sex and closeness of relationship (Misovich, Fisher, and Fisher 1997). Moreover, love, trust, and commitment were used often as reasons for sexual risk-taking, rather than for practicing safer sex (Appleby, Miller, and Rothspan 1999).

Finally, perceived susceptibility to HIV is different for men in relationships versus single men. Men in relationships are more likely to perceive unprotected sex as not risky when it is with a regular partner, as compared to a nonregular partner (Bosga et al. 1995; Bwsse 1998; Lowy and Ross 1994). A study of MSM who were asked how they felt after they had unprotected anal intercourse found that single men were significantly more likely than men in relationships to report feeling worried, scared, and guilty, and were more likely to blame themselves (Hoff, Acree, and Gomez 1999; Hoff and SUMS Team 1999). Another study exploring reasons given by men in relationships who have unprotected sex fell into two general areas; (1) hedonic reasons—for instance, a desire for immediate pleasure, and (2) reasons related to risk estimates, where men describe "pulling out" and "it felt safe with my partner" as strategies for minimizing transmission (Appleby et al. 1999). An explanation for couples having a low perception of risk may be a departure from self-interest toward the "good" of the couple (Drigotas et al. 1999). For example, a partner may believe that in order to be truly intimate (i.e., "good" for the relationship) with his partner, sex must be without a condom.

Method

We conducted a mixed-methods (qualitative and quantitative) study in three phases to: (1) explore relationship issues associated with agreements couples make about sex within and outside the relationship, (2) develop and pilot a quantitative measure focusing on agreements couples make about sex outside the relationship; and (3) test a model of sexual risk-taking for gay male couples. Phase I was a qualitative study in which a series of in-depth interviews was used to explore factors associated with making "agreements about sex" outside the relationship ($N = 45$). In Phase II we developed and pilot tested an "agreements" scale based on data from Phase I ($N = 190$). In Phase III we conducted a cross-sectional study ($N = 566$) combining the new scale and existing measures to develop and test a model of sexual risk for gay male couples.

Case Study—Study Findings

We created a new survey instrument, the Sexual Agreement Investment Scale (SAIS). The items generated to create the scale were based on emergent themes from the qualitative interview data. Themes included: satisfaction with agreement, efficacy of making an agreement, communication about the agreement, how much they valued the agreement, and how committed they were to their agreement. We developed a set of survey items to measure these components of agreements and pilot-tested the items using cognitive interviewing to refine wording and clarity, and then conducted a full pilot study ($N = 380$ gay men, 190 couples). Psychometric analyses extracted a single latent factor, the sexual agreement investment factor, containing 13 items. Internal reliability of the scale was 0.95. Of note, we found that sexual agreement investment was associated with lower odds of breaking the agreement ($OR = 0.81$; 95% $CI = 0.76$, 0.87) and lower odds of engaging in UAI with outside partners of discordant or unknown serostatus ($OR = 0.83$; 95% $CI = 0.76$, 0.89) (Neilands, Chakravarty, Darbes, Beougher, and Hoff 2010). Thus, couples who are more invested in their agreements are less likely to engage in sexual risk with outside partners. This finding opens new avenues for prevention interventions by focusing on teaching couples to make and maintain satisfying agreements.

Using dyadic statistical methods (Kenny 1996) we examined the relationship between interdependence and sexual agreement investment in gay couples. Sums-and-differences dyadic data analyses conducted with concordant negative couples at baseline found a significant effect of the couple-level sum of interdependence on the sum of sexual agreement investment ($N = 266$; B=0.10, $p < .0001$), indicating that couples with higher levels of interdependence had higher levels of investment in their agreements regarding outside sex partners than did couples with lower levels of interdependence. A similar finding was obtained for discordant couples ($N = 99$; B=0.09, $p < .0001$). For concordant negative couples, the within-couple difference in sexual agreement investment between partners was explained by both the couple-level sum ($N = 266$; B=−.02, $p < 0.01$) and couple-level difference ($N = 266$; B=0.03, $p = 0.03$) of interdependence. These results mean that couples with higher levels of interdependence have less discrepancy in their investment in their agreement relative to other couples, and that couples with a greater within-couple discrepancy in interdependence also have greater discrepancies in sexual agreement investment. These findings typify the rich results that are possible to obtain from intact dyads using sophisticated analysis methods such as sums-and-differences and actor-partner analysis.

Conducting this study and developing the SAIS, a scale that is unique to gay couples, was critical to identifying relationship factors associated with risk for HIV. Agreements are a key aspect of gay relationships, and encouraging ongoing communication and maintenance of agreements will help couples reduce risk. Moreover, our ability to conduct dyadic analyses of how couples influence each other's behavior allows us to pinpoint important areas for intervention that are specific to gay couples.

Lessons Learned and Looking Forward

This study contains the largest sample of gay couples in the United States. Totaling all three phases, $N = 801$ couples participated in the study over five years. In order to enroll this many couples into the study, we had to recruit and screen well over 1,500 couples. There were several points in our protocol where we lost couples: We lost some at screening since we screened both partners separately; we lost some at scheduling because we required that they participate at the same time; and we lost many who broke up. Thus, recruiting, screening, interviewing, and surveying couples was time-intensive and expensive. At the time, we designed detailed and labor-intensive protocols to ensure that we were getting the cleanest data possible from both partners of the couple. As mentioned above, understanding how partners influence each other's behavior is critical, but discrepant reports between partners are also important data. For example, 8% of our sample reported discrepant agreement types (i.e., one partner reported a monogamous agreement and one partner reported a nonmonogamous agreement). Clearly, this is an important area in which to intervene in future prevention interventions, and we would not have known that if we hadn't studied both partners. However, in the future, procedures to study and intervene with couples that are less burdensome to staff and participants are needed. For example, developing protocols to recruit and study couples online would be cost-effective, time-efficient, and more convenient for participants. The key is to design protocols that ensure couples are truly couples and minimize dirty data (i.e., partners responding for each other). A next step may be to develop studies that compare existing methods with more efficient and less costly approaches in order to determine with certainty how flexible our methods for studying couples can be. Continuing a rigorous research agenda for the health and well-being of gay couples is essential, and we hope that this study has made a meaningful contribution to that effort.

References

Adib, S. M., Joseph, J. G., Ostrow, D. G., Tal, M., and Schwartz, S. A. (1991). Relapse in sexual behavior among homosexual men: A 2-year follow-up from the Chicago MACS/CCS. *AIDS* 5(6): 757–60.

Appleby, P., Miller, L., and Rothspan, S. (1999). The paradox of trust for male couple: When risking is a part of loving. *Personal Relationships* 6: 81–93.

Arriaga, X. B., and Rusbult, C. E.199. Standing in my partner's shoes: Partner perspective taking and reactions to accommodative dilemmas. *Personality and Social Psychology Bulletin* 24(9): 927–48.

Becker, M. 1974. *The Health Belief Model and Personal Health Behavior*. 2 vols. San Francisco: Society for Public Health Education.

Blumstein, P., and Schwartz, P. 1983. *American Couples: Money, Work, Sex*. New York: William Morrow.

Bosga, M. B., de Wit, J. B., de Vroome, E. M., Houweling, H., Schop, W., and Sandfort, T. 1995. Differences in perception of risk for HIV infection with steady and non-steady partners among homosexual men. *AIDS Education and Prevention*.

Bwsse, A. 1998. Safer sexual decision making in stable and casual relationships: A prototype approach. *Psychology and Health* 13(1): 55–66.

Cáceres, C. F., and Rosasco, A. M. 1997. The correlates of safer behavior among homosexually active men in Lima. *AIDS (London)* 11: S53–59.

Catania, J. A., Kegeles, S. M., and Coates, T. J. 1990. Towards an understanding of risk behavior: An AIDS risk reduction model (ARRM). *Health Education and Behavior* 17(1): 53–72.

Choi, K.-H., Coates, T., Catania, J., Lew, S., and Chow, P. 1995. High HIV risk among gay and Asian and Pacific Islander men in San Francisco. *AIDS* 9(3): 306–8.

Connell, R., Crawford, J., Dowsett, G., Kippax, S., Sinnott, V., Rodden, P., . . . Watson, L. 1990. Danger and context: Unsafe anal sexual practice among homosexual and bisexual men in the AIDS crisis. *Journal of Sociology* 26(2): 187–208.

Davidovich, U., de Wit, J., Albrecht, N., Geskus, R., Stroebe, W., and Coutinho, R. 2001. Increase in the share of steady partners as a source of HIV infection: A 17-year study of seroconversion among gay men. *AIDS* 15(10): 1303–8.

Díaz, R. M., Morales, E. S., Bein, E., Dilán, E., and Rodríguez, R. A. 1999. Predictors of sexual risk in Latino gay/bisexual men: The role of demographic, developmental, social cognitive, and behavioral variables. *Hispanic Journal of Behavioral Sciences* 21(4): 480–501.

Drigotas, S. M., Rusbult, C. E., and Verette, J. 1999. Level of commitment, mutuality of commitment, and couple well-being. *Personal Relationships* 6(3): 389–409.

Ekstrand, M. L., Stall, R. D., Paul, J. P., Osmond, D. H., and Coates, T. J. 1999. Gay men report high rates of unprotected anal sex with partners of unknown or discordant HIV status. *AIDS* 13(12): 1525–33.

Elford, J., Bolding, G., Maguire, M., and Sherr, L. 1999. Sexual risk behaviour among gay men in a relationship. *AIDS* 13(11): 1407–11.

Fishbein, M., and Ajzen, I. 1975. *Belief, Attitude, Intention and Behavior: An Introduction to Theory and Research*. Reading, MA: Addison-Wesley.

Fitzpatrick, R., McLean, J., Dawson, J., Boulton, M., and Hart, G. 1990. Factors influencing condom use in a sample of homosexually active men. *Genitourinary Medicine* 66(5): 346–50.

Goodreau, S. M., Carnegie, N. B., Vittinghoff, E., Lama, J. R., Sanchez, J., Grinsztejn, B., . . . Buchbinder, S. P. 2012. What drives the US and Peruvian HIV epidemics in men who have sex with men (MSM)? *PLoS ONE* 7(11): e50522.

Halkitis, P. N., Wilton, L., Parsons, J. T., and Hoff, C. 2004. Correlates of sexual risk-taking behaviour among HIV seropositive gay men in concordant primary partner relationships. *Psychology, Health and Medicine* 9(1): 99–113.

Harry, J. (1984). *Gay Couples*. New York: Praeger.

Hays, R. B., Kegeles, S. M., and Coates, T. J. 1990. High HIV risk-taking among young gay men. *AIDS* 4(9): 901–8.

Hays, R. B., Kegeles, S. M., and Coates, T. J. 1997. Unprotected sex and HIV risk taking among young gay men within boyfriend relationships. *AIDS Education and Prevention* 9(4): 314–29.

Hoff, C. C. 1998. *HIV prevention among gay male couples*. Paper presented at the AIDS Research Institute Community Presentation Series, San Francisco, CA.

Hoff, C. C., Acree, M., and Gomez, C. 1999. *Gay male couples should be targeted in HIV prevention*. Paper presented at the University-wide AIDS Research Program Annual Investigators' Meeting, San Francisco, CA.

Hoff, C. C., and Beougher, S. 2010. Sexual agreements among gay male couples. *Archives of Sexual Behavior* 39(3): 774–87.

Hoff, C. C., Coates, T. J., Barrett, D. C., Collette, L., and Ekstrand, M. 1996. Differences between gay men in primary relationships and single men: Implications for prevention. *AIDS Education and Prevention* 8(6): 546–59.

Hoff, C. C., Stall, R., Paul, J., Acree, M., Daigle, D., Phillips, K., . . . Coates, T. J. 1997. Differences in Sexual Behavior Among HIV Discordant and Concordant Gay Men in Primary Relationships. *JAIDS: Journal of Acquired Immune Deficiency Syndromes* 14(1): 546–59.

Hoff, C. C., and SUMS Team. 1999. *Sexual risk-taking behavior among HIV+ MSM in primary relationships*. Paper presented at the CDC National HIV Prevention Conference, Atlanta, GA.

Hope, V., and MacArthur, C. 1998. Safer sex and social class: Findings from a study of men using the "gay scene" in the West Midlands Region of the United Kingdom. *AIDS Care* 10(1): 81–88.

Janz, N. K., and Becker, M. H. 1984. The health belief model: A decade later. *Health Education and Behavior* 11(1): 1–47.

Kegeles, S. M., Hays, R. B., and Coates, T. J. 1996. The Mpowerment Project: A community-level HIV prevention intervention for young gay men. *American Journal of Public Health* 86(8, pt. 1): 1129–36.

Kelley, H., and Thibaut, J. 1978. *Interpersonal Relations: A Theory of Interdependence*. New York: Wiley.

Kenny, D. A. 1996. Models of non-independence in dyadic research. *Journal of Social and Personal Relationships* 13(2): 279–94.

Kippax, S., Crawford, J., Davis, M., Rodden, P., and Dowsett, G. 1993. Sustaining safe sex: a longitudinal study of a sample of homosexual men. *AIDS* 7(2): 257–64.

Kippax, S., Noble, J., Prestage, G., Crawford, J., Campbell, D., Baxter, D., and Cooper, D. 1997. Sexual negotiation in the AIDS era: Negotiated safety revisited. *AIDS* 11(2): 191–97.

Lowy, E., and Ross, M. W. 1994. "It'll never happen to me": Gay men's beliefs, perceptions and folk constructions of sexual risk. *AIDS Education and Prevention* 6(6): 467–82.

Martin, J. L., Dean, L., Garcia, M., and Hall, W. 1989. The impact of AIDS on a gay community: Changes in sexual behavior, substance use, and mental health. *American Journal of Community Psychology* 17(3): 269–93.

McKusick, L., Coates, T. J., Morin, S. F., Pollack, L., and Hoff, C. 1990. Longitudinal predictors of reductions in unprotected anal intercourse among gay men in San Francisco: the AIDS Behavioral Research Project. *American Journal of Public Health* 80(8): 978–83.

Misovich, S. J., Fisher, J. D., and Fisher, W. A. 1997. Close relationships and elevated HIV risk behavior: Evidence and possible underlying psychological processes. *Review of General Psychology* 1(1): 72.

Neilands, T. B., Chakravarty, D., Darbes, L. A., Beougher, S. C., and Hoff, C. C. 2010. Development and validation of the sexual agreement investment scale. *Journal of Sex Research* 47(1): 24–37.

Peplau, L. A., Cochran, S. D., and Mays, V. M. 1997. A national survey of the intimate relationships of African American lesbians and gay men: A look at commitment, satisfaction, sexual behavior, and HIV disease. *Psychological Perspectives on Lesbian and Gay Issues* 3: 11–38.

Rempel, J. K., Holmes, J. G., and Zanna, M. P. 1985. Trust in close relationships. *Journal of Personality and Social Psychology* 49(1): 95.

Rusbult, C., and Buunk, B. 1993. Commitment Processes in Close Relationships: An Interdependence Analysis. *Journal of Social and Personal Relationships* 10: 175–204.

Saghir, M. T., and Robins, E. 1973. *Male and Female Homosexuality: A Comprehensive Investigation*. Baltimore: Williams and Wilkins.

Schmidt, K. W., Fouchard, J. R., Krasnik, A., Zoffmann, H., Jacobsen, H. L., and Kreiner, S. 1992. Sexual behaviour related to psycho-social factors in a population of Danish homosexual and bisexual men. *Social Science and Medicine* 34(10): 1119–27.

Stall, R. D., Ekstrand, M., Pollack, L., McKusick, L., and Coates, T. J. 1990. Relapse from safer sex: the next challenge for AIDS prevention efforts. *JAIDS: Journal of Acquired Immune Deficiency Syndromes* 3(12): 1181–87.

Stall, R. D., Hays, R. B., Waldo, C. R., Ekstrand, M., and McFarland, W. 2000. The gay '90s: A review of research in the 1990s on sexual behavior and HIV risk among men who have sex with men. *AIDS (London)* 14: S101.

Sullivan, P. S., Salazar, L., Buchbinder, S., and Sanchez, T. H. 2009. Estimating the proportion of HIV transmissions from main sex partners among men who have sex with men in five US cities. *AIDS* 23(9): 1153–62.

Valdiserri, R. O., Lyter, D., Leviton, L. C., Callahan, C. M., Kingsley, L. A., and Rinaldo, C. R. 1988. Variables influencing condom use in a cohort of gay and bisexual men. *American Journal of Public Health* 78(7): 801–5.

Wieselquist, J., Rusbult, C. E., Foster, C. A., and Agnew, C. R. 1999. Commitment, pro-relationship behavior, and trust in close relationships. *Journal of Personality and Social Psychology* 77(5): 942.

Wu, E., El-Bassel, N., McVinney, L. D., Hess, L., Remien, R. H., Charania, M., and Mansergh, G. 2011. Feasibility and promise of a couple-based HIV/STI preventive intervention for methamphetamine-using, black men who have sex with men. *AIDS and Behavior* 15(8): 1745–54.

PART 3 INTERVENTION DESIGN AND RESEARCH

How Does LGBTQ Health Research Inform Interventions?

José Bauermeister

IMPLEMENTING EFFECTIVE, culturally appropriate public health programs and interventions requires an in-depth understanding of the needs of LGBTQ and other sexual and gender minority individuals. In prior chapters, we explored the importance of theory and research to identify the risk and promotive factors associated with the health and well-being of sexual and gender minority populations. In this section, we provide insights on how to translate research data into the planning and evaluation of LGBTQ health programs and interventions. Given the limited availability of effective interventions to address the various health disparities experienced by LGBTQ communities, the following chapters build on best practices for intervention development and evaluation from the larger public health literature. Rather than proposing a one-size-fits-all approach, however, the authors in this section highlight key considerations to bear in mind when designing, planning, and testing interventions for sexual and gender minority individuals living in diverse contexts. These considerations are crucial to ensure that programs are culturally and contextually responsive to their intended audiences.

Building on the "generations" perspectives that organizes this book, in this section we focus on the empirical and practical considerations related to intervention design and evaluation for LGBTQ communities. Chapter 11 addresses: *Who are you building an intervention for?* and *How does behavior, attraction and identity inform the design of a LGBTQ health intervention?* Rob Stephenson extends the previous discussion of LGBTQ identity in health research (see chapter 4) as it relates to applied (intervention) research. Although the data-collection methods are similar across descriptive and intervention research approaches, their chapter highlights the importance of identifying and characterizing the LGBTQ populations for whom the interventions are being designed. Parallel to prior discussions regarding sampling and data collection in descriptive research, the authors use case studies to illustrate the similarities and contrasts between descriptive research and intervention research. Specifically, the chapter highlights how formative intervention research data (e.g., acceptability, feasibility, and preliminary efficacy) can provide insights into the most suitable research and intervention design, enhance the future intervention's cultural competency, and underscore ethical considerations unique to conducting intervention research for and with LGBTQ populations.

The second chapter in this section, led by Stephen L. Forssell and colleagues, explores the different levels and settings for intervention design and delivery. Building on the socioecological framework discussed in prior chapters, chapter 12 seeks to answer: *What level(s) should an intervention target?* and, accordingly, *What settings might be prime for intervention implementation?* Identifying the appropriate mechanism(s) of change to affect health outcomes in a population is crucial when designing and implementing an intervention for LGBTQ people. Similarly, the setting where the intervention is implemented and rolled out will matter. Through examples, their chapter considers the challenges and opportunities of designing interventions focused at the individual level, within microsystems (e.g., family, school, peers, church), across mesosystems (e.g., interactions between family and teachers or peers) or exosystems (e.g., social services, neighbors, local politics, mass media, industry), and/or affecting macrosystems (i.e., cultural attitudes and ideologies). In discussing these complexities, the authors acknowledge that any attempt to shape behaviors or reduce negative health outcomes through interventions must be informed by, and take advantage of, the multilayered contexts captured by a socioecological framework.

Chapter 13 highlights the importance of community input during the design of an LGBTQ intervention or program. Building on program planning strategies, this chapter asks *What are the some of the community-participatory practices commonly used when developing an intervention?* Recognizing that programs and interventions are most effective when they are informed by a systematic program planning process (McKenzie 2013), José Bauermeister and colleagues describe strategies that may be employed during the intervention planning process to situate an intervention within the specific needs of a community. Using case studies throughout the chapter, the authors emphasize the value and importance of participatory planning processes when seeking to develop health programs for LGBTQ populations and communities.

Chapter 14 focuses on the evaluation and dissemination of interventions. Robin Lin Miller and Angulique Y. Outlaw seek to answer: *How do we evaluate an intervention and decide whether to disseminate and scale it up?* Building on evaluation research paradigms, the authors address the key research issues in moving promising public health and wellness interventions out of the planning and development stages into routine use for the benefit of LGBTQ people. Through a series of examples and case studies, the authors discuss the challenges and opportunities regarding how to transfer a research intervention into day-to-day practice. While intervention efficacy is a vital criterion in evaluation, the authors conclude that practitioners serving LGBTQ communities must ultimately judge whether evidence-supported interventions are effective once institutionalized.

Taken together, we provide a primer on key issues that researchers and practitioners consider when designing and testing LGBTQ health interventions. These chapters can be read independently as an LGBTQ resource or as supplementary readings in courses focused on program planning and evaluation. Given the limited availability of LGBTQ interventions, we hope these chapters elicit your interest in intervention development and evaluation in your future work.

ELEVEN

Engaging Populations in LGBTQ Health Interventions

Rob Stephenson and Erin Riley

IN THIS chapter, we expand on previous discussions of LGBTQ identity and health to explore ways in which identity must be considered when designing research, with a particular emphasis on the considerations for designing intervention research. The chapter begins with an overview of identity definitions through a research-focused lens and continues to explore the research design, cultural awareness, and ethical considerations that must be made when designing and conducting intervention research with LGBTQ populations. Case studies are provided to illuminate the issues that may arise.

Understanding Identity

The terms *gender* and *sex* are often conflated and used interchangeably without question (Cameron 2005). Sell and Conron describe the meanings and history of these terms in chapter 4, and it is useful to revisit those definitions here as a foundation for discussing research design and conduct considerations. *Sex* refers to sexual anatomy, physiology, genetics, and hormones; while *gender* is a psychological, social, and legal construct (Egan and Perry 2001). The terms *male*, *female*, and *intersex* are categories that describe sex. Terms like *woman, man, cisgender, transgender, genderqueer,* and so on describe gender.

Sex Assigned at Birth

At birth, individuals are typically classified on a birth certificate as male or female based on physical appearance. The phrase "sex assigned at birth" (Mayer et al. 2008) is used to recognize that the sex label was "assigned" to an individual that may not reflect their current identity or biology. When conducting intervention research with LGBTQ populations, we may want to focus on research that is most relevant to a specific sex. For example, we may be interested in cervical cancer prevention in the LGBTQ community. An intervention focused on cervical health would be limited to individuals who have a cervix. In order to ensure that our intervention reaches participants who meet the anatomical criteria, we may want to recruit and screen our participants based on their sex assigned at birth, rather than their current gender identity.

Gender Identity

Gender identity is how individuals defines themselves, typically as a man, woman, a mixture of both, or something else. Gender identity may be the same or different from one's sex assigned at birth (Holmes and Meyer-hoff 2008). There may be times when, as researchers, we want to explore an intervention research question for those with a specific gender identity. For example, we may be interested in improving primary health care use among LGBTQ women. In contrast to the cervical health example described earlier, the use of primary health care is not restricted to individuals with specific physical characteristics. Therefore, for the women's primary health care intervention, we may want to use current gender identity as an eligibility criterion, rather than recruit and screen our participants based on anatomy or sex assigned at birth. This would allow us to include all those who identify as women in our research study.

Let's pause and consider how the two previous examples relate to intervention design and recruitment. In the cervical health example, we were interested in only those who had a cervix. By screening based on anatomy, our sample may include individuals who were assigned female at birth and who may have any current gender identity. In the primary health care example, we were interested only in those who currently identify as women; therefore our sample may include any individual who currently identifies as a woman regardless of what sex they were assigned at birth. There may also be times when we want to specifically focus our research on the transgender community: those for whom their current gender identity is different from their sex assigned at birth. For intervention research that specifically focus on transgender populations, it is necessary to include both sex assigned at birth and current gender identity as a means of identifying transgender participants. This is referred to as the "two-step process" and comprises questions on both sex assigned at birth and current gender identity (see chapter 4 for details).

Gender Expression

Gender expression is the way in which people express their gender identity through their behavior, clothing, ways of speech, and other outward forms of expression (Morrow 2006). Individuals may use names and personal pronouns to expresses their gender as well (Hildalgo et al. 2013). Gender expression can be any combination of masculine, feminine, and androgynous traits (Morrow 2006). Someone may express their gender is ways that do not conform to expectations of their sex or gender identity. In designing interventions and intervention research, it is important not to conflate gender identity and gender expression. For example, when designing a study for transgender women, a potential participant may present with what the research staff perceive as a masculine gender expression. However, if that person identifies as a woman, they meet that eligibility criterion, regardless of gender expression.

Sexual Orientation

As defined in chapter 4, sexual orientation refers to romantic or sexual attraction, behavior, and identity. It is important to note that gender does not denote sexual orientation. Cisgender and transgender people may have any sexual orientation. Therefore, it is important to separate gender and sexual orientation questions when conducting research. Sex assigned at birth, current gender identity, and current sexual orientation should be distinct and separate questions.

Sexual and Gender Minority Groups

A sexual minority is someone who has a sexual orientation that differs from what is most common in society (Mayer et al. 2008). Gender minorities include people who have a gender that differs from their sex assigned at birth. The National Institutes of Health Sexual and Gender Minority Research Office includes individuals with intersex conditions and/or differences of sex development (DSD) under the umbrella of gender minorities. When conducting research among the broad group of sexual and gender minorities, it is important to assess sex assigned at birth, gender identity, history of intersex/DSD, and multiple aspects of sexual orientation (e.g., attraction, behavior, and identity).

Some individuals or groups do not identify with LGBTQ terminology. For example, in one research study, participants preferred to identify as men who have sex with men (MSM) rather than *gay* because they felt the term *gay* was associated with elite, Western ideals (Boellstroff 2011). In another research study, men who reported engaging in same-sex behaviors and were not born in the United States did not describe themselves as *gay* because the word does not exist in their native language or their sexual orientation was not rigidly categorized (Zea et al. 2003; Wolitski et al. 2006). There is a risk that individuals who do not identify as LGBTQ may be excluded from intervention research if the questions used to assess gender identity or sexual orientation have response categories that do not reflect their experience. For example, a question assessing sexual orientation that includes only asks about identity categories (e.g., lesbian, gay, bisexual) and not about behavior (e.g., same-sex partners) may miss a significant proportion of sexual minorities. Studies specifically assessing sexual orientation identity may include an "other" option for participants to write in their sexual orientation identity, and/

or list as many response options as possible. The latter requires extensive knowledge of terminology used in the population of interest and benefits from formative qualitative work with the community to identify the range of labels used to describe sexual orientations.

Of course, sex, gender, and sexual orientation do not make up the entirety of an individual's identity. A person will hold multiple identities and ways of representing themselves to the world (Meyer and Northridge 2007). For example, someone at a party is unlikely to introduce herself only as "a lesbian." She may be more likely to describe her likes, dislikes, origin, political affiliation, religion, or interests. Each of these makes up her identity. As scientists conducting research with, and proposing interventions for, LGBTQ populations, it is essential to consider multiple aspects of an individual's identity that may be salient to the research topic.

Designing and Implementing Intervention Research with and for the LGBTQ Community

Let's now turn our attention to how to design and conduct intervention research studies that are simultaneously respectful of identities and also facilitate the accurate capture of both identity and behavior. The first issue to consider is the use of language and terminology when conducting LGBTQ-focused intervention research; the use of this language should be considered throughout the research—from design to recruitment to delivery of the intervention. The language we employ and the labels we apply to people must be thought through with sensitivity and respect. Individuals should be able to choose how others refer to them. It is important not to assume that we know which labels someone prefers, or whether they use labels at all. The use of labels that the participant or potential participant does not identify with may be perceived as offensive and deter study participation. While it is respectful to allow our target community to self-identify and create their own labels, we must also have a clearly defined set of eligibility criteria to ensure enrollment of appropriate participants into a research study. There is no one way to approach this, and there is no singular correct way to use terminology. Preferred language and terminology may vary by context: geographical location, race and ethnicity, age, or multiple other factors. Interventionists should take the time to work with the community to understand the preferred language and terminology within that community prior to gathering data to inform their intervention, design a program, and recruit participants for their intervention trial. Researchers conducting LGBTQ-focused intervention research need to be cognizant of the harm that can be created through misuse of language and should not dismiss the labels and language preferred by potential participants as "simply semantics."

Insider or Outsider Participation

Another consideration for researchers embarking on LGBTQ intervention research is the extent to which they also belong to or identify with the LGBTQ community. Even researchers who themselves have an LGBTQ identity should be aware that their identity doesn't necessarily confer access to or understanding of all LGBTQ communities. Contextual variations should be considered when working with a specific community or set of communities (Bettinger 2008; Bettinger 2010). When planning intervention research with LGBTQ communities, it is important to consider whether one is considered an "insider" or "outsider" to the community, and to understand the logistical and ethical issues associated with each. An LGBTQ-identifying researcher conducting LGBTQ intervention research may be seen as an insider, and as a member of the community they may have greater knowledge of the community and greater cultural sensitivity around language and other issues. An LGBTQ researcher may be knowledgeable about venues from which to recruit LGBTQ participants or have access to key community stakeholders who may be important in introducing the research to the community. Knowing that the researcher is LGBTQ-identifying may reduce discomfort among research participants, although Bettinger (2010) argues that shared LGBTQ-identity alone is not enough to dissolve discomfort, and that there are other important researcher- and context-specific characteristics (e.g., age, race) that could equally shape the level of participant discomfort. It is never appropriate to pretend to have an LGBTQ identity in order to gain access to an LGBTQ community for research. Many researchers work with communities with identities that differ from their own. The most important approach is to work with LGBTQ communities in a respectful, ethical, and sensitive manner.

Ethical Considerations

A guiding principle of all research is that it is conducted ethically and does no harm to the research subjects involved. In addition to the general ethnical principles of respect for persons, beneficence, and justice, it has been suggested that there are additional ethical considerations when conducting research with LGBTQ populations. In many settings, same-sex behavior and/or "cross-dressing" is illegal. Even in settings where it is not illegal, stigma and discrimination are common. LGBTQ populations are often therefore socially and economically marginalized, with increased risk of violence, police harassment, and exploitation. Given this vulnerability, there is a potential for participants to be harmed by participation in the research. Intervention research with LGBTQ populations must therefore take precautions to prevent these harms.

LGBTQ participants may require special protections around confidentiality (Radford 1998). If an intervention study is advertised as a LGBTQ study or is widely known locally to be for LGBTQ individuals, a participant may face significant risks of undesired disclosure of their sexual orientation or gender identity. This may also introduce bias into the study, if only those who feel comfortable as identifying as LGBTQ in that setting are willing to participate. To reduce these risks, researchers may want to use non-LGBTQ-specific names and images to promote the study. It may be a risk for the participant to have a copy of a signed informed consent form for others to find. Therefore researchers should consider seeking a waiver of written consent, opting instead for oral consent; or, if written consent is required, not requiring the participant take a copy of the consent form with them.

Researchers should also consider how they communicate with their participants for retention. For example, leaving a voicemail about a LGBTQ health program may risk disclosure to others who hear the message. Seeking permissions from participants to contact them, having them choose a preferred method of contact (text/SMS, voice mail, email), and having them choose a preferred message (e.g., "we are calling about your health study involvement") are all ways to protect and respect participants.

Harm may arise during data collection as well. Asking about same-sex behaviors or gender identity in settings where such identities and behaviors have been stigmatized and/or punished may pose the risk of significant discomfort or emotional distress to participants. Ensuring that participants know they can refuse to answer any questions is a vital part of the informed consent process, and LGBTQ participants must be reassured that they can refuse to answer questions without consequence and that data they provide will be kept confidential. Researchers should also screen for and monitor signs of emotional distress and have the appropriate referral systems in place to refer participants who are in need of help.

Regardless of the identity of the researcher, one should be aware of their own potential for heterosexist and cisgender-centric bias—for example, allowing for only "man" or "woman" as response options for gender risks, omitting sectors of the community who do not identify within this binary. Being faced with invisibility or exclusion in this way may anger, frustrate, or offend the potential participant, causing them emotional harm, and it may also harm the relationship between the researcher, the individual, and the community. Thus, it is essential to ensure that data collection instruments are as inclusive as possible for the research topic.

The history of research that pathologizes LGBTQ communities has facilitated mistrust of research among some members of the LGBTQ community (Herek et al. 1999). In his review of LGBTQ research methodologies, Bettinger (2010) cites Martin and Meezan (2003), who discuss the "ample history of medical and social science research involving LGBT populations that have violated contemporary ethical standards" (p. 183), and they provide examples ranging from lack of informed consent and invasion of privacy to castration to "cure" homosexuality. While these studies obviously harmed individuals, other studies created prejudice against LGBTQ communities by promoting negative stereotypes (Herek 1998). The resultant mistrust and suspicion of research in some LGBTQ communities must thus be considered when designing and implementing intervention research. It is imperative that members of the LGBTQ community be included in the research process from inception to dissemination. Creating research projects that are LGBTQ-focused without the involvement of LGBTQ community members risks the perception that researchers are taking data from the LGBTQ community for their own purposes and not for the express good of the community. It also risks the research not being culturally appropriate and aligned with and respectful of the needs of the community.

Designing, Recruiting, and Implementing LGBTQ Intervention Research

In this section, we examine the practical considerations of designing intervention research focused on LGBTQ populations. We use case studies to explore the practical and ethical considerations of balancing scientific needs and cultural sensitivity.

Descriptive Research

Scientists may choose to use a descriptive research study design to understand a population prior to developing an intervention (Kothari 2004). Descriptive research answers questions such as "what, why and how" for a population being studied and does not seek to create change within a population (Elbogen 2002). Descriptive research may be qualitative or quantitative in nature. Qualitative descriptive studies may collect and analyze qualitative data in order to understand perceptions, attitudes, or norms. Let us consider the example of a study that wants to examine the experience of intimate partner violence among gay men. The study hypothesizes that gay men may experience higher rates of violence in their relationships due to the social stressors they experience as members of a sexual minority group. In order to test this hypothesis, the research study must recruit and collect data from men who identify as gay. If such a study were to recruit based on behavior (e.g., MSM), then the study risks asking questions that are not relevant to participants who do not identify as gay. Let us consider two case studies:

CASE STUDY 1

In 2012, a descriptive research study took place in Atlanta, Georgia, to examine the prevalence of intimate partner violence among gay and bisexual men, as well as the associations between experiencing homophobia and experiencing violence. The study recruited by placing advertisements in local gay-themed newspapers, publications, and flyers in local gay-themed venues. Flyers contained images of male couples in intimate poses—holding hands and hugging—to send the message that this was a study for male couples. The advertisement also included the heading *"Gay Male Couples Study—Join Now!"*

CASE STUDY 2

In 2012, another descriptive research study took place in Atlanta, Georgia, to examine attitudes toward HIV testing among young MSM. The goals of the study were to collect qualitative data to understand the barriers that MSM faced when seeking HIV testing. The study recruited by placing advertisements in local gay-themed newspapers and venues, and also in non-gay-themed venues and publications. The advertisements included images of a single young man, and included the heading *"Young Men's Health Study—Join Now!"*

Let us consider the differences between these two case studies. Some are obvious. Case study 1 is quantitative and is recruiting couples; case study 2 is qualitative and is recruiting men regardless of relationship status. Additionally, the differences in the aims of the two studies mean that the desired study populations are very different: case study 1 wants to recruit men with a particular sexual orientation identity, and case study 2 wants to recruit men based on their sexual behavior and not their identity. The approaches to recruitment are thus different. In case study 1, greater accuracy in recruitment can be achieved by using the word *gay* in the recruitment materials to purposively select those with that identity. Case study 2 is attempting to recruit men who have sex with men. Including *MSM* on the advertisement material could have several negative effects: alienating members of the gay community who do not want their identity reduced to sex and alienating men who, although they may have sex with men, do not feel comfortable with an MSM label. Using a generic and nonoffensive research project title allows the research to cast a wide net for recruitment. Once potential participants approach the research team, they can be screened for eligibility by asking questions on sexual behavior. In these examples, we see how we can balance the need to recruit those with a particular identity or behavior with the need to respect the community and avoid creating selection bias in our samples.

Intervention Research

Intervention research is concerned with developing and testing an intervention to create change around a predetermined attitude, behavior, or clinical measure in a specific population. A clear and simple definition for the study population is essential. Failing to accurately define the study population may lead to bias in the research by sampling people who either do not fit the eligibility criteria or cannot experience the outcomes under observation. As an illustration, think back to the earlier example of studying cervical health in the LGBTQ community. If we developed an intervention to prevent cervical cancer, we would want to ensure that we tested its impact only among those who were at risk of experiencing cervical cancer, i.e., people who have a cervix. Hence, we would want to be sure that our eligibility criteria were specific. Relying exclusively on gender identity to recruit may result in a bias if women (cisgender or transgender) who did not have a cervix were included in the sample. Below we consider eligibility definitions for LGBTQ research at the individual and couple (dyadic) levels.

Individual

Desired characteristics of the individual participants should be aligned with the research goals and hypothesis; that is, if the goal is to assess smoking behavior among lesbian women, then the eligibility criteria must consider both gender and sexual orientation. If the goal is to look specifically at stigma among transgender women, regardless of their sexual orientation, then the eligibility criteria need to assess sex assigned at birth and gender identity. Identifying the boundaries and characteristics of the study population is a critical first stage in the research design. This will ensure that the correct population is recruited and that the intervention is tested with the correct group.

CASE STUDY 3

A recent research study aimed to increase HIV testing among transgender youth between the ages of 15 and 24. In eligibility screening materials, the two-step process was used in which a question was asked about sex assigned at birth and was followed by a question on current gender identity. Researchers give participants a choice of gender identities, including transgender, trans masculine, trans feminine, male, female, or other. This allowed broad recruitment of those whose current gender identity was different from their sex assigned at birth and also ensured that participants felt respected and empowered to name their own identity. This is particularly important for intervention research. The success of intervention research rests on the ability to recruit and retain participants with whom you will test the efficacy of the intervention. Ensuring respect for identity in the recruitment phase is key for creating a positive environment for the individual, and it can have a significant impact on the retention.

Couples

There has been a recent growth in research interest in the health of same-sex couples. The term *same-sex couple*, rather than gay or lesbian couple, recognizes that two people with the same sex are in a romantic or sexual relationship and does not take into account sexual orientation identities. As is the case with designing intervention studies that focus on individuals, intervention studies that focus on couples must also have clear eligibility criteria and employ recruitment techniques that are both accurate and sensitive. The eligibility criteria should match the goals and hypotheses of the study: for example, if the study is specifically interested in the lived experiences of lesbian couples, then criteria must include both gender and sexual orientation identity. The other consideration is whether there needs to be concordance in identities between the couple. That is, do both members of the couple need to have the same gender and sexual identity? For a study of the lived experiences of lesbian couples, the answer would probably be yes. But for a study that wanted to develop an intervention to improve condom use among MSM couples and that wanted to intervene with both men, then it would not be necessary for them to have concordance in sexual orientation identities. One man may identify as gay and the other as straight, but as long as they reported concordance in sexual behavior, then they would be eligible for the study. Recruiting and working requires defining what constitutes a couple. There is no standard definition of a couple. For some it is about emotional attachment, for others it is co-residence, and for others sexual exclusivity. Many intervention studies allow couples to self-define. That is, many research studies ask questions about relationship type (e.g., partner, spouse) and duration of relationship. But the central question when recruiting couples to LGBTQ-focused intervention work is the extent to which the individual and joint identities of the couple are expected to shape the success of the intervention.

Recruitment Based on Study Research Questions

Perhaps the biggest challenge for researchers when developing interventions for LGBTQ-populations is to have a narrow definition of the study population that allows a specific hypothesis about the effect of an intervention to be tested. In order to achieve this, researchers must understand concepts of intersectionality and the fluidity of identity.

Challenges of Defining Populations in Terms of One Identity

It is essential that researchers recruit participants in a way that considers intersecting identities. Researchers must decide which identities matter for answering their research question. For intervention research, this means deciding what the intervention target is: is it focused on a behavior regardless of identity (e.g., increasing HIV testing), or is it focused on shifting behavior among a particular gender and/or sexual orientation? Once this is answered, researchers must then develop their recruitment and screening materials in a way that allows the appropriate study population to be identified and not alienate others. Below we show some examples.

Figures 11.1 and 11.2 are both examples of banner advertisements that are used to recruit same-sex couples into research studies (on the left a study of male couples, on the right a study of female couples). Notice that words are sparse in the recruitment materials. No identity is listed or attributed to either of the couples. But the imagery, through the intimate portrayal of two people, makes it clear that these are two people involved in an intimate realtionship. These are banner advertisements, and so potential participants would click on these ads and be taken to a survey where they would be screened for eligibility. These ads are likely to attract people who have same-sex attraction or sexual behavior even if they identify as LGBTQ, and they are also likely to attract same-sex couples who identify as gay, bisexual, or lesbian. Both of these studies intended to recruit a range of same-sex couples, regardless of sexual orientation. If sexual orientation were the required criterion, then that could have been messaged in the advertisement.

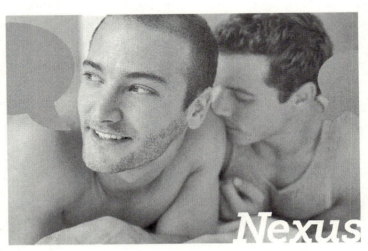

Figure 11.1. Recruitment image for study of male couple's health

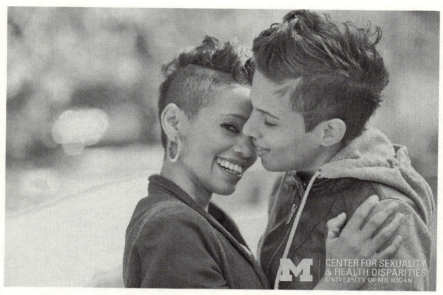

Figure 11.2. Recruitment image for study of sexual minority health

Identity Fluidity

Another challenge for researchers recruiting LGBTQ participants is that identities may change over time. One way to address this issue in observational descriptive studies is to repeat measures. For developing and testing interventions, researchers must also ask whether fluidity matters to the success of their intervention—that is, does it matter whether participants change their identity over time? This may mean that a particular participant passes in and out of a predetermined eligible population. In these cases, it may make the most sense to have identity criteria at recruitment and screening and have those criteria measured throughout the timeframe of the intervention but not lead to study ineligibility, once enrolled.

Reluctance to Self-identify as LGBTQ

Sexual practices, gender identity, and sexual orientation are sensitive topics that may be addressed in LGBTQ research. Potential participants may fear stigma and discrimination and may thus be reluctant to participate or refuse to answer specific questions. This could lead to underreporting or nonresponse biases. During recruitment, researchers should ensure that participant data will be kept safe and confidential and that privacy is maintained (Dillman, Symth, Christian, and Dillman 2009). Additionally, researchers should involve individuals drawn from the desired study population to ensure that recruitment materials are culturally appropriate and acceptable. These issues highlight the importance of involving the LGBTQ community in the inception, design, and implementation of intervention research, which will not only increase acceptability but also decrease data bias.

Online Recruitment

Online recruitment for LGBTQ intervention research is common. Online recruitment allows researchers to access potential participants who may not be reachable in person (Riggle, Rostosky, and Reedy 2005) and has the potential to be less costly and more efficient than recruitment through physical venues. While there are benefits to using online recruitment methods, there are also some challenges. Race and class biases inherent in online research have been well documented. It is difficult to retain participants for studies without the use of incentives, which may be challenging to distribute online (Riggle, Rostosky, and Reedy 2005). Additionally, it is more difficult to prove whether the online participant is a real person or whether they are conducting fraudulent scams (Graham et al. 2011). However, recent guidelines have been developed and published that describe methodologies for detecting and reducing fraud among online research studies (Teitcher et al. 2015).

Time-Location Sampling

Sampling frames are rarely available in LGBTQ research. That is, there is no complete list of people who identify as LGBTQ. One approach to this problem has been to create a sampling frame that is composed of venues from which you may be able to recruit LGBTQ individuals. From this sampling frame, time-location sampling is used to recruit a sample of the population of interest. The creation of the sampling frame starts by interviewing members of the population of interest to identify a list of locations or specific times to recruit potential participants into research studies (Gallagher et al. 2007). This can be done through focus group discussions with community members or through interviews with community leaders. In addition, a researcher with insider knowledge may be able to start the list on their own and add to that list with community input. Involving the community in developing a list of LGBTQ venues is a good way to reduce bias in the identification of venues. It is imperative that those designing the list of venues represent the intended study population. For example, if the research aims to recruit young African American gay men, then the researcher needs to ensure that the people making the list of venues are young African American gay men. It is also important to regularly update the list of venues used for sampling. Regularly checking in with the community to update the list of venues ensures that the sampling frame remains relevant and accurate and that the community knows that you are paying attention.

Conclusions

This chapter has explored some of the ethical, cultural, and practical considerations that are necessary when designing and implementing research with and for LGBTQ populations. We purposefully use the phrase *with and for* the LGBTQ community throughout this chapter to recognize two important points. *Science is with the community*: engagement of the community throughout the research process is vital for improving both cultural sensitivity and scientific accuracy. *Science is for the community*: the aim of research should be to generate new knowledge and to do no harm, and thus special protections are often needed when working with the LGBTQ community to ensure that their well-being and confidentiality are upheld. This chapter has provided practical examples of how this can be achieved, and has provided recommendations for ensuring that a balance of scientific rigor and cultural sensitivity is achieved.

References

Ahmed, S. 2006. *Queer Phenomenology: Orientations, Objects, Others*. Durham, NC: Duke University Press.

Ahmed, S. F., Morrison, S., and Hughes, I. A. 2004. Intersex and gender assignment: The third way? *Archives of Disease in Childhood* 89(9): 847–50.

Bettinger, T. V. 2007. Gay men at midlife and adult learning: An uneasy truce with heteronormativity. In L. Servage and T. Fenwick, eds., *Proceedings of the Joint International Conference of the 48th Annual Adult Education Research Conference and the 26th Annual Canadian Association for the Study of Adult Education*, 43–48. Halifax, Nova Scotia: Mount Saint Vincent University.

Bettinger, T. V. 2008. "You know what I'm saying": Emic and etic considerations in research involving sexual minorities. In S. L. Lundry and E. P. Isaac, eds., *Proceedings of the 49th Adult Education Research Conference*, 9–13. St. Louis: University of Missouri.

Bettinger, T. V. 2010. Ethical and methodological complexities in research involving sexual minorities. *New Horizons in Adult Education and Human Resource Development* 24(1): 43–58.

Boellstorff, T. 2011. "But do not identify as gay": A proleptic genealogy of the MSM category." *Cultural Anthropology* 26(2): 287–312.

Cameron, D. 2005. Language, gender, and sexuality: Current issues and new directions. *Applied Linguistics* 26(4): 482–502.

Conron, K. J., Scout, and Austin, S. B. 2008. "Everyone has a right to, like, check their box": Findings on a measure of gender identity from a cognitive testing study with adolescents. *Journal of LGBT Health Research* 4(1): 1–9.

Dillman, D. A., Smyth, J. D., Christian, L. M., and Dillman, D. A. 2009. *Internet, Mail, and Mixed-Mode Surveys: The Tailored Design Method*. Hoboken, NJ: Wiley & Sons.

Egan, S. K., and Perry, D. G. 2001. Gender identity: A multidimensional analysis with implications for psychosocial adjustment. *Developmental Psychology* 37(4): 451–63.

Elbogen, E. B. 2002. The process of violence risk assessment: A review of descriptive research. *Aggression and Violent Behavior* 7(6): 591–604.

Eliason, M. J., Dibble, S. L., Gordon, R., and Soliz, G. B. 2012. The last drag: An evaluation of an LGBT-specific smoking intervention. *Journal of Homosexuality* 59(6): 864–78.

Fish, J. 2008. Navigating queer street: Researching the intersections of lesbian, gay, bisexual and trans (LGBT) identities in health research. *Sociological Research Online* 13(1): 104–15

Gallagher, K.M., Sullivan, P.S., Lansky, A.k, and Onorato, I. M. 2007. Behavioral surveillance among people at risk for HIV infection in the US: the National HIV Behavioral Surveillance System. *Public Health Reports* 122 (supp. 1): 32–38.

Graham, R., Berkowitz, B., Blum, R., Bockting, W., Bradford, J., de Vries, B., . . . and Makadon, H. (2011). *The Health of Lesbian, Gay, Bisexual, and Transgender People: Building a Foundation for Better Understanding*. Washington, DC: Institute of Medicine.

Grant, J. M., Mottet, L. A., Tanis, J., Herman, J. L., Harrison, J., and Keisling, M. 2010. *National Transgender Discrimination Survey Report on Health and Health*

Care. Washington, DC: National Center for Transgender Equality and the National Gay and Lesbian Task Force.

Greene, G. J., Fisher, K. A., Kuper, L., Andrews, R., and Mustanski, B. 2015. "Is this normal? Is this not normal? There is no set example": Sexual health intervention preferences of LGBT youth in romantic relationships. *Sexuality Research and Social Policy* 12(1): 1–14.

Herek, G. M., Gillis, J. R., and Cogan, J. C. 1999. Psychological sequelae of hate-crime victimization among lesbian, gay, and bisexual adults. *Journal of Consulting and Clinical Psychology* 67(6): 945–51.

Herek, G. M. 1998. Bad science in the service of stigma: A critique of the Cameron group's survey studies. In G. M. Herek, ed., *Psychological Perspectives on Lesbian and Gay Issues* 4: 223–55. Thousand Oaks, CA: Sage.

Hidalgo, M. A., Ehrensaft, D., Tishelman, A. C., Clark, L. F., Garofalo, R., Rosenthal, S. M., . . . and Olson, J. 2013. The gender affirmative model: What we know and what we aim to learn. *Human Development* 56(5): 285–90.

Holmes, J., and Meyerhoff, M., eds. 2008. *The Handbook of Language and Gender*. New York: John Wiley & Sons.

Kothari, C. R. 2004. *Research Methodology: Methods and Techniques*. New Delhi: New Age International.

Martin, J. I., and Meezan, W. 2003. Applying ethical standards to research and evaluations involving lesbian, gay, bisexual, and transgender populations. In W. Meezan and J. I. Martin, eds., *Research Methods with Gay, Lesbian, Bisexual, and Transgender Populations*, 181–201. New York: Harrington Park Press.

Mayer, K. H., Bradford, J. B., Makadon, H. J., Stall, R., Goldhammer, H., and Landers, S. 2008. Sexual and gender minority health: What we know and what needs to be done. *American Journal of Public Health* 98(6): 989–95.

Meyer, I. H., and Northridge, M. E. 2007. *The Health of Sexual Minorities*. New York: Springer.

Morrow, D. F. 2006. Sexual orientation and gender identity expression. In D.F. Morrow and L. Messingers, eds., *Sexual Orientation and Gender Expression in Social Work Practice: Working with Gay, Lesbian, Bisexual, and Transgender People*, 3–17. New York: Columbia University Press.

Pike, K. L. 1990. On the emics and etics of Pike and Harris. In R. G. Headland and M. McClelland, eds., *Emics and Etics: The Insider/Outsider Debate*, 28–47. Newbury Park, CA: Sage

Radford, J., ed. 1998. *Gender and Choice in Education and Occupation*. New York: Routledge.

Reisner, S. L., Biello, K., Rosenberger, J. G., Austin, S. B., Haneuse, S., Perez-Brumer, A., . . . Mimiaga, M. J. 2014. Using a two-step method to measure transgender identity in Latin America/the Caribbean, Portugal, and Spain. *Archives of Sexual Behavior* 43(8): 1503–1514.

Riggle, E. D., Rostosky, S. S., and Reedy, C. S. 2005. Online surveys for BGLT research: Issues and techniques. *Journal of Homosexuality* 49(2): 1–21.

Schippers, M. 2007. Recovering the feminine other: Masculinity, femininity, and gender hegemony. *Theory and Society* 36(1): 85–102.

Teitcher J. E. F., Bockting W. O., Bauermeister J. A., Hoefer C. J., Miner M. H., and Klitzman, R. L. 2015. Detecting, preventing, and responding to "fraudsters" in internet research: Ethics and tradeoffs. *Journal of Law and Medical Ethics* 43(1): 116–33.

Wolitski, R. J., Jones, K. T., Wasserman, J. L., and Smith, J. C. 2006. Self-identification as "down low" among men who have sex with men (MSM) from 12 US cities. *AIDS and Behavior* 10(5): 519–29.

Zea, M. C., Reisen, C. A., and Díaz, R. M. 2003. Methodological issues in research on sexual behavior with Latino gay and bisexual men. *American Journal of Community Psychology* 31(3–4): 281–91.

TWELVE

Finding the Right Approach for Interventions with LGBTQ Populations

Stephen L. Forssell, Peter Gamache, and Rita Dwan

HEALTH PRACTITIONERS must not presume that singular approaches are effective for the populations that they seek to help. This principle is especially important for developing health interventions for LGBTQ populations. Elsewhere in this volume, we have considered the critical importance of having a solid understanding of the socioecological framework that envelops our population of interest. Bronfenbrenner (1979, 1986) was among the first to posit a model that considers human development in the context of the individual (e.g., sex, age, health), microsystems (e.g., family, school, peers, church), mesosystems (e.g., interactions between family and teachers or peers), exosystems (e.g., social services, neighbors, local politics, mass media, industry), and macrosystems (i.e., cultural attitudes and ideologies). An understanding of these complexities provides an operative guiding principle that allows us to form models of the social determinants of health and that acknowledges that individuals do not experience health developments in isolation. Any attempt to shape behaviors or attitudes through interventions must be informed by and take advantage of the multilayered contexts captured by a socioecological framework. Specifically, the model can inform how best to:

1. Develop an understanding of and effectively recruit intervention participants;
2. Discover the contexts for optimal delivery of an intervention; and
3. Identify appropriate mechanisms of change for that population.

Understanding and Recruiting Diverse LGBTQ Populations

The aim of this section is to convey the importance of fully understanding the characteristics, norms, and values of a population of interest in order to effectively recruit and retain LGBTQ participants into a health intervention. Often, implementing an existing intervention requires additional adaptation prior to its use with a new population or context. Merely changing placeholders for gender identity or sexual orientation generally will not work. For instance, an obesity intervention that has been demonstrated to be efficacious with heterosexual Latina women cannot necessarily be assumed to gain the attention, buy-in, and participation of lesbian African American women. Thus, understanding your health intervention goals within the context of your specific LGBTQ population is vital.

Getting to Know Your Population: Best Practices and Approaches

Taking a "community-involved" approach helps secure buy-in from the population you are seeking to impact and assists in both effective intervention design and recruitment of participants. Participatory approaches such as community-based participatory research (CBPR) strive to make partnerships with the populations of interest in order to address health disparities (Wallerstein and Duran 2006). By design, CBPR engages stakeholders in the intervention development, implementation, and evaluation process. While an admittedly time-consuming process, this approach can pay dividends by capitalizing on the unique perspectives of community members and local organizational representatives, creating more culturally competent and successful interventions.

A number of tools can be used in a community-involved intervention development. Focus groups of seven to ten individuals can be effective at identifying key characteristics of the target population (Greenbaum, 1998). The benefit of focus groups is that because of their interactive nature, they help identify nuanced qualitative characteristics of the population that do not arise from single-respondent quantitative surveys or even open-ended written responses or individual interviews. A drawback is that they are relatively expensive to conduct, and usually more than one focus group is recommended in order to obtain a complete picture of the intervention population. Importantly, unlike surveys or other measures that are intended to be representative of the population as a whole, focus groups should represent a narrow subset of the target population, and the participants should be as alike as possible, since participants in focus groups are more willing to engage openly and honestly when among similar others (Greenbaum 1998). Similarly, these smaller subgroups may have unique characteristics that are not discoverable in mixed groups. For instance, if your intervention seeks to reduce rates of smoking in Latino LGBTQ communities, you might want to conduct separate focus groups for lesbian and bi women, gay and bi men, and transgender persons—perhaps broken up by age cohort, depending on the size and nature of your particular population and your intervention objectives. In this way focus groups give you a window into the particular characteristics of the subgroups that make up the whole of your population.

Peer ethnography is a related approach that involves gathering information through direct observation and face-to-face social interaction with members of the target population in order to gain a holistic view of that community (Mutchler, McKay, McDavitt, and Gordon 2013). Similar to focus groups, peer ethnographers come from the target population and provide first-hand accounts and other information about that population. Unlike focus groups, peer ethnographers are recruited and interviewed individually and are trained to make observations and take field notes about the population and behaviors within the community. The use of gatekeepers, or frontline health professionals or lay people as informants about the community of interest, is another tool that can be used effectively in your approach to intervention design. Gatekeepers can inform a living intervention about how it is being received by participants, enabling adjustments and redirection if needed (Skerret and Mars 2014, Teo et al. 2016).

Web-based applications and social media have become widely used and effective tools for reaching a population of interest, both to explore and understand a population, and to recruit participants for interventions. They can be especially helpful in connecting with geographically and culturally isolated individuals and to reach ethnic minorities in health studies (Couper 2000; Hirshfield, Grov et al. 2015; Martinez, Wu, Shultz, Capote, Rios, Sandfort, and Rhodes 2014). Web-based tools can also provide a cost-effective alternative to in-person focus groups. Video conference- or webinar-based focus groups can yield useful information, but the depth of in-person interactions and nonverbal information (facial expressions, hand gestures) is considerably restricted. Participants are also more likely to be distracted or less involved in "e-focus groups" than in in-person settings.

Recognizing Diversity across LGBTQ Populations during Intervention Development

There are myriad differences *within* the LGBTQ community to consider in the intervention process. Perhaps the most important caveat is to avoid falling victim to the fallacy of the unified, monolithic community. That is, there is no such thing as *the* LGBTQ population or *the* LGBTQ community. Lesbian, gay, bisexual, and transgender individuals share many social, cultural, and political interests in common, yet these constituencies can be radically different when it comes to individual health behaviors that we are trying to impact. Interventions aimed at reducing risky sexual activity, for example, should take into account that some studies have found sexual behaviors of behaviorally homosexual men to differ from those of behaviorally bisexual men with respect to the number of sexual partners (Jeffries 2011) and baseline risky sexual behaviors (Smalley, Warren, and Barefoot 2016). Support-seeking differences that could affect health and health behaviors might also exist. For example, Frost and colleagues (2016) found that gay and bisexual men in their study were more likely to rely on other LGB people and on chosen families, whereas lesbian participants tended to rely more on their families of origin (Frost, Meyer, and Schwartz 2016).

Differences also exist between transgender and cisgender lesbian women, gay men, and bisexual individuals regarding interactions with and attitudes about care providers (Institute of Medicine 2011; Kitts 2010). It is well established that LGBTQ persons report receiving poorer-quality medical care than cisgender heterosexual people (Institute of Medicine 2011). Furthermore, transgender people report significantly more barriers to care and more negative experiences with care providers than lesbian, gay, or bisexual patients (Lambda Legal 2010; Macapagal, Bhatia and Greene 2016). Additionally, questioning and queer-identified patients have reported more negative experiences with care providers than gay, lesbian, and bisexual patients (Macapagal, Bhatia, and Greene 2016). Potential transgender, queer, and questioning intervention participants might be expected to approach health or medical interventions with greater skepticism. To counteract potential objections or hesitance, your intervention marketing and messaging might want to acknowledge this distrust and provide reassurances that these participants will be treated with respect by culturally competent professionals.

Recruitment Considerations

As a general rule, it is advisable to recruit participants from various sources (Hartlieb, Jacques-Tiura, Naar-King, Ellis, Catherine Jen, and Marshall, 2015). A multipronged recruitment strategy prevents intervention groups from becoming too homogenous, maximizes the chance of reaching as many in the target population as possible, and increases the opportunities to tap into diverse social networks within the population. Known within-community differences should be addressed in your recruitment plan. If your intervention is aimed at improving communication between same-sex male and female partners, for example, recruitment should consider that coupled lesbian women tend to live in more rural areas than gay male couples (Kazyak 2012). Additionally, although gay men and lesbians hold many social and political interests in common, the two groups also tend to maintain different social networks (Esterberg 1996).

Convenience sampling (CS) is the most commonly used approach for obtaining participants. However, CS is infamously less representative than alternative approaches designed to reach specialized populations or for greater generalizability. Time-space sampling (TSS) and respondent-driven sampling (RDS) are two such alternatives for recruitment in hard-to-reach or at-risk populations. TSS is a systematic sampling approach focusing on venues (such as nightclubs) identified through community mapping frequented by a target population. RDS, on the other hand, capitalizes on social networks of a population of interest (Clark et al. 2014; Forrest, Stevenson, et al. 2014). RDS studies have revealed that social networks often spread out in spider web–like fashion across cities and larger geographical regions (e.g., Magnus et al. 2013). In contrast with traditional "snowballing," which is vulnerable to volunteer bias, RDS intervention participants refer a given number of other participants directly into the intervention in a systematic manner. The RDS strategy is a particularly helpful, though time-consuming, tool for penetrating hard-to-reach social networks (Bryant 2014; Clark et al. 2014; Tourangeau, Edwards, Johnson, Wolter, and Bates 2014).

Recruitment and intervention materials must also acknowledge that not all sexual and gender minority individuals embrace the categorical labels and associations laid out by the initials L, G, B, and T. For instance, consider the task of reducing HIV transmission in behaviorally bisexual men. Reaching out to support groups for men who identify as bisexual may entirely miss those who self-identify as heterosexual but engage in sex with men discreetly (Zule, Bobashev, Wechsberg, Costenbader, and Coomes 2009). Similarly, many who prefer to identify as queer reject labels of lesbian, gay, or bisexual and might not be responsive to recruitment messaging and behavior change efforts targeted in that way. Furthermore, with regard to sexual orientation, those who identify as queer or pansexual might have different risk profiles than peers who identify as gay, lesbian, or bisexual in behaviors as varied as drug use, diet, unprotected sexual activity, driving without a seat belt, and likelihood to seek medical care (Smalley, Warren, and Barefoot

2016). Gender-queer or gender nonbinary persons may not respond to messaging aimed at the trans community that assumes a gender binary. Including terms such as transmen and transwomen or acronyms such as F2M and M2F in marketing materials without appealing to nonbinary-identified trans people could alienate and exclude many that you may wish to include in your intervention population. Furthermore, differences in health risk behaviors have been found between nonbinary and transgender men that could be important to take into account in your approach (Smalley, Warren, and Barefoot 2016). In these instances, reaching out separately to these groups with language that incorporates resonant terminology and buzzwords could bolster recruitment and retention.

LGBTQ individuals also vary in the degree to which they identify with and accept cultural norms surrounding the dominant LGBTQ experience. The literature is replete with research and interventions that enroll participants from gay-affirming organizations and events, such as Pride festivals, bars and restaurants in predominantly gay neighborhoods, or through homophile organizations (e.g., Grov, Rendina, and Parsons 2014; Kimmel, Rose and David, 2006; Pantaloneet al. 2010). While this is an effective approach for obtaining a large convenience sample, a significant subset of the target population that does not frequent these institutions or perhaps even use the term *gay* as a self-label, is missed. LGBTQ people who live in rural areas or in more socially conservative environments, for instance, typically have less access to or feel less connected to "mainstream" LGBTQ culture and the accompanying gay establishments and Pride events (Garnets and Kimmel 2003). To address these challenges, it may be necessary to minimize the strength of the connection to a dominant gay culture in both the messaging and the distribution of recruitment materials in order to address the sensibilities of a population or subset of a population less embedded in "out" LGBTQ culture. For example, in a dyadic intervention for LGBTQ cancer survivors and their caregivers, Kamen, McMahon, Heckler, Heffner, Morrow, Mustian, and Bowen (2016) discovered that some participants reacted negatively to the use of *LGBT* in the title of the study and in a promotional brochure. Ultimately, the researchers edited brochures and flyers to remove *LGBT* from the study title and description to avoid unintentionally broadcasting the sexual orientation or gender identity of potential participants. Consider also that early in the response to the AIDS crisis, researchers learned to use terminology that targeted the risky behavior, i.e., "men who have sex with men" (MSM), rather than identities (for example, "gay men") that appealed to those more deeply embedded in urban gay culture.

Intersectionality, or the focus on the importance of multiple interlocking marginalized identities, has become a critical consideration in research, in clinical practice, and for designing health interventions for LGBTQ populations (Bowleg and Bauer 2016; Ng 2016; Rosenthal 2016). Intersectional approaches require us to consider the layered social and cultural influences on the person in the context of broader systems of power and oppression, not just their individual sexual orientation and gender identity in isolation. In this framework race, ethnicity, social class, and culture are considered as diverse, complex, and intertwined sources of identities that relate to diverse norms, values, and behavior.

For the intervention to have its intended effect, your recruitment approach must consider this intersection of separately marginalized identities and demonstrate an understanding of the populations' circumstances. Different cultures may view the labels of *gay* and *lesbian* as constructs that do not apply to their experiences. Many Asian cultures, for instance, see *gay* and *lesbian* as American or Western ideological constructs that are learned or voluntarily embraced rather than as innate identities (Chan 1995). Developing recruitment materials that contain imagery and language that are both culturally competent and relevant to the communities of interest is essential. Furthermore, in the presence of stigma and discrimination, ensuring the protection of participants' privacy is also critical, both as communicated in recruitment materials and as practiced in the intervention process. Ideally, in-person interactions with participants should occur at locations that are both discreet and accessible by public transportation. Offering travel vouchers and flexible evening and weekend appointment hours can improve retention and reduce missed appointments. Similarly, acknowledging the historical incidence of mistreatment of African American and transgender persons by medical professionals and researchers, and assuring participants that they will be provided with competent and respectful treatment and care, can go a long way toward improving recruitment and retention (Nation 2016).

Intervention Contexts: Health Intervention Settings

A critical determination of any intervention approach is the setting in which the intervention is to occur. Numerous contexts and settings can be considered for the delivery of your health intervention at various points along the socioecological map. Here we present seven different settings for interventions: online; in homes, schools, and workplaces; and in partnership with community-based organizations, clinics, and churches.

Online Health Interventions

Internet-based interventions have the clear advantage of offering participants privacy and a feeling of anonymity, thus increasing some individuals' willingness to participate. For LGBTQ people, privacy can be crucial, particularly within communities with high degrees of rejection or violence toward LGBTQ individuals. Online interventions also have the potential to reach a broad number of individuals cheaply and quickly. A distinct disadvantage of the approach, however, is that participants may feel free to falsify their responses in a more anonymous and private setting.

Mustanski, Greene, Ryan, and Whitton (2015) effectively capitalized on an online delivery method to promote sexual health among LGBTQ youth. Their Queer Sex Ed (QSE) intervention delivered sexual health information online to 202 LGBTQ youth ages 16–20. Narrated text, anatomical images, and videos were used to educate participants, and health-related content included topics such as how to make sex pleasurable, communicate health needs in a relationship, and reduce risks. Mustanski and colleagues (2015) evaluated specific aspects of QSE, including the feasibility of enrolling LGBTQ youth into an online sexual health intervention, the acceptability of and engagement with the intervention, and the efficacy of the online intervention. Participants rated the QSE intervention positively and were engaged with its internet-based delivery. The average time participants spent with the content exceeded 90 minutes, demonstrating that they devoted time to learning the material. Comparisons between participants' responses to assessments before and after the intervention revealed a significant improvement in knowledge of sexual functioning, STIs, HIV, HIV testing, contraceptive methods, and risk of transmitting STIs through certain sexual behaviors.

As the availability, affordability, and capabilities of technology increase, the future of health interventions will certainly include not only more website-based online platforms but also other electronic modalities such as biomedical monitoring devices and smart phone apps (Doyle-Lindrud 2014; Kirby and Thornber-Dunwell 2014) for participant interaction, data collection, and health education.

Home-Based Health Interventions

Home-based intervention settings have the ability to reach more comprehensively into participants' daily lives, holding the capacity for tremendously positive impact. However, the particular environment where each participant lives must be fully understood, especially for LGBTQ people. Family members' negative attitudes about sexual orientation and gender identity can significantly affect how a family member avoids LGBTQ discussions. Alternately, family members who affirm LGBTQ identity can be an important source of support for a successful intervention. Additionally, the intervention itself must be maintained over an extended time period for it to create sustained behavioral change. "One-off" home-based interventions are not likely to produce lasting effects. As such, the design and implementation of home-based interventions are necessarily time-intensive and potentially costly. That said, carefully designed and well-funded longitudinal home-based interventions have considerable potential.

Few home-based interventions with LGBTQ populations have been examined rigorously in the literature. However, one intervention program aimed at improving family relationships for LGBTQ youth in the home provides an example of the potential power of home-based approaches, as well as the need to understand family dynamics. The Family Acceptance Project is an initiative developed at San Francisco State University (Ryan and Chen-Hayes 2013). From in-depth interviews with 245 LGB young adults ages 21–25, Family Acceptance Project researchers documented the negative impact of parental rejection as a response to a child's coming out as L, G, B, or T (Ryan, Huebner, Diaz, and Sanchez 2009). They also provided evidence for protective effects of an accepting reaction on the part of parents (Reitman, Austin, et al. 2013; Ryan, Russell, et al. 2010). From these findings, they developed trainings that honored the social and religious diversity of the families they were serving. They provided videos and other materials in English, Spanish, and Chinese aimed at encouraging parents to support their LGBTQ children in the home.

There is much more that could be accomplished through home-based interventions to positively impact the lives of LGBTQ people in the future. By targeting family dynamics and support systems, home-based interventions could be used to impact domains such as romantic partner relationship quality, parenting skills, domestic violence, and substance abuse. Moreover, subjecting these interventions to rigorous evaluation and peer review would add to a relatively sparse body of literature on evidence-based practices in the LGBTQ population.

School-Based Health Interventions

Schools are potentially powerful venues for implementing interventions for LGBTQ youth. Schools and school systems offer the advantage of having large groups of same-aged peers gathered together on a regular basis and an infrastructure to assist with the delivery of an intervention. Particularly salient goals for interventions within schools are the reduction of stigma, depression, and anxiety among LGBTQ youth, and the reduction of bullying and homophobia among peers. Across the country, however, one will find vastly different attitudes and concomitant policies in primary and secondary school systems not only about LGBTQ-related topics, but about sexuality and sexual health in general (Holmes and Cahill 2004). School systems and individual schools have, to varying degrees, initiated or engaged with interventions aimed at creating a safe space for students to study and socialize, reduce stigma and harassment, and foster a more accepting environment for LGBTQ youth (Meyer and Bayer 2013). Thus, obtaining buy-in from individual school systems, administrators, teachers, and parents is essential (Meyer and Bayer 2013).

One of the earliest school-based efforts to reduce stigma and harassment of LGBTQ students was Project 10 in Los Angeles. Project 10 was founded in 1984 by Virginia Uribe at Fairfax High School in the Los Angeles Unified School District. It was the original model for school-based LGBTQ Youth interventions that followed, having endured much resistance throughout its creation more than 35 years ago (Quintanilla 1989). The Friends of Project 10 organization (http://friendsofproject10 .org/) maintains resources for educators seeking to create similar intervention programs. In other cases, special magnet schools such as the Harvey Milk School in New York were specifically created to provide safe and productive environments for LGBTQ students who were not succeeding in traditional school environments. Gay-Straight Alliances (GSAs) as support mechanisms for LGBTQ youth have flourished across the country in recent years (Poteat, Scheer, et al. 2015; Russell, Muraco, et al. 2009), and can serve as community stakeholders and entry points for school-based intervention.

There is clearly much more to be accomplished to support LGBTQ youth and decrease bullying and discrimination against them by their peers. Future school-based interventions to support LGBTQ students should continue to focus on the issues critical to these youth—stigma, depression, bullying, and homophobia—and reach into regions of the country that are underserved. The relative dearth of a body of methodologically rigorous literature on school LGBTQ programs also suggests that it is advisable to model future school-based interventions on existing evidence-based interventions in schools (see Borum and Verhaagen 2006).

Workplace Health Interventions

As LGBTQ employees become increasingly visible in the workforce, employers are paying more attention to their LGBTQ employees by adapting more supportive policies. The business case for inclusion and diversity is grounded in the assumption that employees who can be comfortably out in the workplace feel safer and happier, making them healthier and more productive. At the same time, workplace discrimination has been demonstrated to have a deleterious effect on the health of LGBTQ persons (Bauermeister, Meanley, Hickok, Pingel, VanHemert, and Loveluck 2014; Nadal 2011). Furthermore, workplace discrimination against LGBTQ employees can impede career advancement and create hostile work environments (Beatty and Kirby 2006). These observations clearly outline the advantages of workplace interventions to improve the health of LGBTQ employees. More progressive corporations have heeded these findings and engage in diversity training aimed at reducing stigma and harassment of their LGBTQ employees. According to the Human Rights Campaign, 52% of Fortune 500 companies offer sensitivity training on sexual orientation issues, while 42% offer training on gender identity (HRC 2016).

However, despite numerous motivating factors for employers to adopt such programs, there is still resistance in some work environments to implementing interventions to improve LGBTQ workers' work environment. Reasons behind inaction include local sociocultural norms resistant to supporting LGBTQ people, both within the corporate structure and in the broader community, the lack of equal protection for LGBTQ workers in many states, and even laws or policies that explicitly discriminate against LGBTQ people in employment and public accommodation (Lambda Legal 2017). Barron and Hebl (2011), for instance, reviewed the state of workplace protections for LGBTQ people and found a mixed bag of legal protections, leaving private employers in many states free to discriminate or to allow discrimination and harassing situations to continue unabated.

At the time of this writing, we could not identify any published peer-reviewed examples of workplace interventions specifically oriented to LGBTQ workers. Much of what has been developed in this area is proprietary and not available publicly. However, Hunt and colleagues reviewed existing interventions related to the reduction of workplace sexual harassment (Hunt, Davidson, Fielden and Hoel 2010). They offered a Sexual Harassment Intervention Model based on extant interventions involving management commitment to explicit antiharassment policies and multiple levels for intervening, including at a primary level (e.g., trainings, evaluations, employee empowerment), a secondary level (complaints procedures), and a tertiary level (rehabilitation). Hunt and colleagues' paradigm, or similar workplace interventions, could be used as models for future LGBTQ workplace interventions. An effort should be made to publish evidence-based models for workforce interventions specifically on LGBTQ employee issues. This could benefit smaller companies without the resources to hire outside firms to implement worker training programs and interventions.

Community-Based Health Interventions

Community-based organizations (CBOs) are a frequent context for health interventions with the LGBTQ community. They are in many ways ideal settings for conducting an intervention. Generally speaking, CBOs are inherently co-invested in positive outcomes for LGBTQ clients. Community-based interventions overall have the advantage of capitalizing on community networks and the infrastructure of existing community groups to design, inform, and implement an intervention effort through community-based participatory research or other approaches. Depending on the community partners and stakeholders one works with, community-based interventions can be critical in reaching specific racial and ethnic groups of interest. Challenges to community-based interventions can include managing the scope necessary to successfully reach into a community population and, of course, the accompanying costs involved in larger-scale interventions. A community approach is also limited by whatever access one has to community members and organizations with the willingness and resources to participate. Rural areas and smaller cities, for instance, may have fewer organized community groups with which to partner.

One notable example of a successful community-based intervention was the HOLA program (Sun, García, Mann, Alonzo, Eng, and Rhodes 2015). HOLA was a lay health advisor intervention targeting the reduction of HIV infection rates among Latino gay and bisexual men and other MSM, as well as transgender persons in the United States. Sun and colleagues recruited participants from the community to serve as lay health advisors or *Navegantes*. Each of the eleven Navegantes selected were trained in HIV reduction techniques, and each recruited eight nonoverlapping members of their social networks who were also gay, bisexual, other MSM, or transgender to participate in the intervention. Over the course of one year, the Navegantes held meetings and facilitated various activities that were designed to promote sexual health among the enrolled participants. Activities included condom distribution, discussions about sexual health, referrals to health centers, and screening of videos about HIV, STDs, and condom negotiation. Sun and colleagues collected process evaluation data of intervention implementation from the eleven Navegantes, documenting 1,820 activities, most commonly condom distribution, with community members. They also found that their prevention messages were ultimately delivered not just to the eight primary contacts, but also to other community members. The HOLA intervention provides evidence for the broad reach of lay health advisor approaches and of the value of the community-based participatory research approach.

Based on a growing body of evidence of the efficacy of community-based participatory research (Northridge, McGrath and Krueger 2007; Wallerstein and Duran 2006), in the future we can look to community-based health interventions to address untapped and still-emerging domains of LGBTQ health in order to reduce disparities and improve the availability of culturally competent care. As rural and more traditionally conservative regions of the country see greater numbers of out LGBTQ people, opportunities for reaching out to LGBTQ community members and establishing partnerships to support the health of the population will arise. It will be critical to capitalize on these openings as they emerge.

Clinic-Based Health Interventions

Clinical settings are another common contact point for intervening in the health of LGBTQ persons. Clinics are designed to be able to meet with and treat high volumes of clients and patients, providing a preexisting mechanism for interacting with intervention participants. Interventions in clinic settings, large and small, have been developed and implemented to address myriad issues such as the physical and mental health of LGBTQ elders (Hash et al. 2013) and gay fathers (Barret 1996), safer sex and HIV prevention (e.g., Bluespruce et al. 2000; Wanigaratne, Billington, and Williams 1997), and HIV serostatus disclosure (Przybyla 2010). Limitations of conducting interventions in clinical settings, as with community-based interventions, include challenges with managing the size, scope, and cost of an intervention. Additionally, clinics in more rural and socially conservative areas may be less likely to have LGBTQ-specific services or established connections with LGBTQ populations, or the resources and willingness to sponsor an intervention with LGBTQ clients.

One clinically based intervention (Thurston, Bogart, Wachman, Closson, Skeer, and Mimiaga 2014) addressed the problematic issue of adherence to HIV medication protocols in HIV-positive LGB youth. HIV treatment adherence is critical to control of the effects and spread of HIV, but it can be difficult to maintain, even for adults. Treatment adherence in youth can be particularly challenging. Thurston et al. (2014) developed a technology-enhanced HIV treatment adherence intervention targeting LGB adolescents and young adults for use in clinical settings. Their five-session intervention, named *Positive STEPS* (Positive Strategies to Enhance Problem Solving) employed cognitive-behavioral and motivational interviewing techniques as methods for encouraging behavioral change in HIV-infected youth. These five sessions, led by masters- and doctoral-level clinicians, involved customized problem-solving strategies to help youth confront adherence barriers including poor risk perception about consequences of non-adherence, seeing medication as a reminder of HIV status, irregular daily schedules, lack of social support, poor mental health, medication side effects, nondisclosure of HIV status, opposition to medical instructions, complicated medication regimens, fatigue from chronicity of HIV, balancing transition to managing their own HIV care, self-blame, shame, and stigma. Their published study (Thurston et al. 2014) reported on two case descriptions of individual intervention participants during the intervention and at follow-up.

In the future we can look to clinical settings to continue to be a viable means of reaching LGBTQ intervention populations. As with community-based intervention efforts, expanded visibility of LGBTQ people in rural and more conservative geographical areas will provide opportunities for clinics to directly reach out to and serve LGBTQ community members. Interventionists should be ready to establish partnerships with clinics that support these underserved populations.

Health Interventions in Churches and Other Places of Worship

This is a currently expanding area, ripe for exploration by interventionists. Religious institutions are traditionally seen as less accepting of LGBTQ individuals than the public at large. Those religious traditions whose teachings present more negative imagery of LGBTQ people and same-sex sexual behavior have more negative impacts on the mental health, identity development, and resiliency of developing LGBTQ persons (Gibbs and Goldbach 2015; Walker and Longmire-Avital 2013; Wolff, Himes, Soares and Miller Kwon 2016). LGBTQ-identified adherents of religious institutions, particularly more socially conservative ones, may be less likely to be connected to LGBTQ organizations in mainstream society and more likely to be closeted. Interventions in religious settings could therefore offer access to a subset of the LGBTQ population not reached in other contexts. Furthermore, churches and other places of worship could be productive settings for reducing homophobia and discrimination against LGBTQ people found in socially conservative faith communities. A disadvantage of working in these settings, therefore, might be resistance to interventions aimed at supporting LGBTQ people and changing negative attitudes about them.

Given the stigma surrounding an LGBTQ identity and issues of sexuality in general in many faith communities, it is perhaps unsurprising that there is little in the published literature on faith-based interventions with the LGBTQ population. Church-based and other faith-based interventions have, however, recently been used to address health issues such as diabetes (Timmons 2015) and smoking cessation (Schoenberg, Bundy, Bispo, Studts, Shelton and Fields 2015). A growing number of church-based HIV interventions are being developed and implemented. Molock, Zea, Risen, and Poppen (unpublished manuscript), for instance, are working with Black churches in Washington, DC, to develop a pilot study and intervention aimed at assessing the extent of HIV risk behaviors in adolescents who have religious affiliations and to identify factors that would promote effective linkages to care. In a similar intervention, Abara, Coleman, Fairchild, Gaddist, and White (2015) employed a faith-based model aimed at building capacity in African American churches in South Carolina to assist them in successfully developing, implementing, and sustaining locally developed HIV/AIDS prevention interventions.

Future interventions with faith communities will need to expand into areas more directly supportive of LGBTQ participants in areas other than sexual risk behaviors. Despite steps forward on HIV interventions in churches, few faith-based HIV interventions explicitly include gay men, MSM, and transgender individuals within their designs. Fewer still address other crucial areas of concern to LGBTQ-identified people in faith-based settings, such as positive identity development, mental health, risk for suicide, discrimination, stigma, and homophobia. There is potentially much to be gained from identifying allies in religious communities, particularly those from historically less supportive denominations and traditions, to intervene with more positive messaging about LGBTQ identities and sexual behavioral health messages.

Identifying Appropriate Mechanisms of Change

We have surveyed seven specific settings for implementing interventions with the LGBTQ population. Yet across these varied contexts, the actual behavioral change mechanism can be found at any one of five levels that reflect the systems embedded in the socioecological model. What do we mean by *mechanisms of change*? The mechanism of change is the actual mode of interaction between interventionist and participant in which the behavioral or attitudinal modification occurs. Identifying the appropriate mechanism or mechanisms is a critical decision. Selecting the appropriate mechanism can make the difference between a successful intervention and one that misses the mark. In the following section, we identify five mechanisms through which health interventions occur: at the level of the *individual*, through *dyadic* interactions, through *small group* interactions, through *community-level* interactions, and, most broadly at the level of *structural and policy* changes. Regardless of the mechanism, interventions ultimately aim to affect the behavior and health outcomes of individuals. We will briefly describe each mechanism, its strengths and weaknesses, and provide examples of its use with LGBTQ populations.

Individual: Behavioral, Biomedical, and Combination Interventions

Individual behavioral interventions seek to change the health-related cognitions and behaviors of individual persons through interactions with single intervention participants. Although published studies measure the effectiveness of health interventions on many individuals, they target each person separately and measure the effectiveness of the intervention. Individual-level interventions may do so through face-to-face in-person sessions, or remotely through the internet or web- or app-based tools. Approaches employed in these contexts commonly involve engagement of participants through independent, self-guided learning and through interactions with clinicians, peer educators, audiovisual tools, or computer-assisted self-interviews. One obvious benefit of this approach is that the intervention can be personalized, at least to some degree, to meet the challenges or needs of the person participating. It can also give the person participating a sense of individual attention and perhaps a greater assurance of confidentiality. For those reasons, the individual mechanism of change can be effective in highly personal and private behavior change such as sexual behaviors or in HIV prevention. A drawback is that the overall process can be long and expensive, particularly if the intervention population is a large one. The previously mentioned Queer Sex Ed (QSE) intervention (Mustanski et al. 2015) is one such example of an intervention based on an individual-level mechanism of change employed with a LGBTQ population. In the QSE intervention, individual participants interacted with online materials including videos aimed at reducing sexual risk and improving sexual communication, as well as making sex more pleasurable.

In addition to behavioral change, individual-level interventions can be designed to have a biomedical impact on a population. For instance, biomedical interventions in medical, clinical, and public health settings have been found to be effective in moderating biological and physiological factors to prevent HIV infection and reduce susceptibility to HIV, including the promotion of the use of pre-exposure prophylaxis or "PrEP" (Beyrer 2015) and improved adherence to anti-retroviral medication protocols (HIV/AIDS Prevention Research Synthesis Project).

Dyadic: Couples, Patient-Provider

Certain health issues are better addressed by targeting pairs of individuals. This dyadic mechanism addresses one or both individuals who are part of a two-person relationship. The relationship could be, for instance, that of a romantic couple, a patient and their health provider, or a parent and child. Where the target of the intervention is one specific person in the dyad, the second person, presumably interpersonally close to the target individual, helps facilitate the intervention or provides support and motivation. Alternately, the mechanism may attempt to change the dynamic between both individuals in a relationship, such as one that targets communication between sexual partners or family members. Common strategies for dyadic interventions include couple counseling, interviews, facilitated discussion and role play, and seminars and presentations (e.g., Grant, Anderson, McMahan, Liu, Mico, Hosel et al. 2014; Montgomery, Watts and Pool 2012; Szabo, Whitlatch, Orsulic-Jeras, and Johnson 2016). The obvious strength of a dyadic approach is its ability to have an impact with couples or other two-person relationships. In some cases, dyadic approaches may be adaptable to three- or more person relationships. Otherwise, their impact is limited to pairs of individuals.

Fals-Steward, O'Farrell, and Lam (2009) reported promising results of an alcohol-use disorder intervention for lesbian couples. This intervention was designed to help women in a lesbian relationship decrease the number of days they spent drinking alcohol heavily. It did so by including both lesbian partners, wherein one was struggling with alcohol use problems while the other was not. Elements of the longitudinal intervention included abstinence goal setting and partner support. The intervention sessions were facilitated by lesbian women or women in same-sex relationships and took place in a gay and lesbian health center. The control group targeted only individuals and employed education on maintaining abstinence. Although there was a significant decrease in the percentage of days participants engaged in heavy drinking in both the control and intervention groups, only the intervention group showed a significant decrease in heavy drinking one year later.

In the previous section we discussed both behavioral and biomedical interventions in the context of the individual-level mechanism of change. In some situations, it is optimal to incorporate a combination of behavioral and biomedical approaches. Persons' behaviors around initiating or adhering to medical treatment protocols are a prime example of such fertile ground for combination interventions. One particular combination medical/behavioral intervention that employed a dyadic mechanism of change was conducted by Martinez, Wu, Levine, Muñoz-Laboy, Fernandez, and Bass et al. (2016). They adapted an evidence-based behavioral intervention called Connect 'n Unite (CNU), previously used successfully with substance-using Black male couples to reduce HIV risk behaviors. Martinez and colleagues added a biomedical component to the CNU intervention, specifically education about pre- and post-exposure prophylaxis (PrEP and PEP). Through a series of focus groups conducted with Latino MSM in New York City recruited through social media and apps such as Grindr, the interventionists further adapted the protocol to be culturally competent and relevant with Latino MSM and their male partners. The intervention comprised informational sessions addressing communication and support within relationships, strategies for self-care, education about HIV/AIDS and risk behaviors, and information about PrEP and PEP as tools for prevention of the spread of HIV. After the intervention, participants expressed a desire for information about these biomedical interventions, in particular requesting that PrEP and HIV self-testing kits be made available to them.

Small Group: Family, Support Groups

Interventionists have also facilitated health behavior change through small group mechanisms. Generally, this mechanism tries to influence outcomes of individuals within a group by taking advantage of the interdependent or supportive dynamic of the group. Members of families and support groups, for example, possess common interests and health concerns, and have a level of commitment to assisting and supporting one another. Commonly used small group intervention strategies include class-based instruction and group counseling, group exercises, and facilitated role play. This approach capitalizes on the strength of the interpersonal relationships in the targeted groups, though this can be limited in effectiveness if group members are not supportive of each other. Rizer, Mauery, Haynes, Couser, and Gruman (2015) conducted a systematic literature review of interventions for LGBTQ men and women and identified three successful small group interventions that were used to provide support and incentives to affect specifically targeted behaviors such as smoking cessation, breast self-examination, and mammogram screening (Bowen, Powers and Greenlee 2006; Eliason, Dibble, Gordon and Soliz 2012; Walls and Wisneski 2011). These interventions each employed techniques that attempted to increase peer support and education about behavior change and were led by a trained member of the LGBTQ community.

Community: Psychological Empowerment, Community Capacity

In contrast to small group mechanisms, a community-level mechanism of change looks to have effects on a broader scale. This mechanism attempts to permeate a community with common challenges as broadly as possible with health messages aimed at improving outcomes for community members. "Train-the-trainer"–style interventions, for instance, are designed to reach directly into a specific subset of a community and identify individuals who will serve as agents of change among others in their community in order to have a broader community-level impact than individual small group interventions can have. Small group exercises, brainstorming sessions, facilitated discussions, and report-back breakout sessions are common activities and strategies for engaging participants. The community-level mechanism has the advantage of potentially reaching a large group of individuals, with the capacity to influence norms of behavior. The drawback of this approach is that it requires substantial resources in the form of trainers and materials in order to reach a scope that can have an impact. Community-based interventions are often conducted in multiple cities or jurisdictions, requiring building cooperative relationships over a broad geographical area. One such example of an effective train-the-trainer intervention was the Leadership in Advocacy and Planning (LEAP) program (Thompson, Forssell, and Wunder 2008), a project of the Ryan White Comprehensive AIDS Resources and Emergency (CARE) Act. LEAP was a three-day training program that offered persons living with HIV/AIDS opportunities to become involved in Ryan White–related advisory and planning groups. It also offered persons already involved with Ryan White programs additional training and education on how CARE Act groups operate, as well as information about how to organize HIV/AIDS prevention-related activities within trainees' home communities. Trainings were held at two pilot sites in Washington, DC, and Chicago. Subsequent revisions were made to the program content, and an additional 14 trainings were conducted across the country. A total of 245 individuals completed the LEAP training over the course of a year. Onsite evaluation instruments were administered, and three- and six-month follow-up assessments were conducted through a telephone-based, structured interview. The results from the evaluation of LEAP indicated that the program had a positive impact on graduates' HIV/AIDS-related community activities. Participants reported using aspects of the training in their subsequent professional and advocacy activities. Moreover, HIV/AIDS activities were sustained and increased over the follow-up period for a significant minority of LEAP graduates.

Structural and Policy-Based Mechanisms

The broadest domain of mechanism of change is at the policy or structural level. This mechanism attempts to influence the institutions that make decisions about the health-related structures they control with the goal of making those institutional structures more impactful and effective. Along with community-level mechanisms, policy-level mechanisms hold the greatest potential for most directly impacting the social determinants of health. Policy-driven interventions can vary widely in size and scope. When we think of policy, we often "think big," such as in federal or state government. For that reason, the strength of a policy or structural intervention is its potential for sweeping and permanent change that could perhaps affect thousands of individuals. The challenges embedded in these types of interventions are gaining buy-in from a diverse group of stakeholders and navigating the political landscape within the domain of interest.

A readily available example of federal-level structural change related to the health of LGBTQ people was the introduction of the 2010 Patient Protection and Affordable Care Act (ACA). The legislation mandated the creation of health insurance exchanges in states across the country to make health insurance policies available to those who previously could not afford them. Moreover, the initiative included efforts specifically targeted at the LGBTQ population. Out2Enroll is a marketing campaign and web-based resource rolled out in tandem with the launch of ACA exchanges, designed to encourage LGBTQ people to purchase health care plans through the insurance marketplaces set up by the ACA (http://out2enroll.org/). Research indicates that both the broader ACA effort and the Out2Enroll campaign have been successful at increasing the percentage of the general population and of the LGBTQ population that have health insurance (Baker, McGovern, Gruberg, and Cray 2016).

Bear in mind that "Big P" policy initiatives at the federal or state level are not the only policy-based opportunities to affect positive health changes. "Little p" policy, such that can be enacted at the level of a small organization, medical facility, clinic, or private practice, can also be a conduit for mechanisms of behavioral health change. A hospital, for instance, can adopt and mandate LGBTQ cultural competency training for its staff. Or a primary care medical practice might revise its intake forms and electronic medical record-keeping protocols to make them sensitive to nonheterosexual relationship status and the gender diversity of its patients.

One specific structural intervention conducted in Taiwan exemplifies how "little p" policy can have a significant impact on health behaviors. Ko and colleagues (Ko, Lee, Hung, Chang, Lee, Chang, and . . . Ko 2009) evaluated a structural intervention aimed at reducing unprotected sexual contact and increasing condom accessibility in gay bathhouses in three Taiwanese cities. Using a quasi-experimental design, nine bathhouses were observed as either control condition locations or intervention locations where free condoms were provided and bathhouse attendees were invited to complete a questionnaire and to be screened for HIV and other STIs. In a follow-up study, 270 participants were surveyed at six months post-intervention, finding that intervention participants were more likely to report accessing condoms inside bathhouses than those attending control bathhouses. Likewise, condoms were more likely to be available at the reception desk of the bathhouse entrance.

As with any policy-driven effort, a clear drawback of this mechanism is that what can be done can be undone. As has been made clear in recent efforts to repeal the ACA, policy can be both adopted and reversed.

Conclusions

Interventions designed in consultation with the socioecological context of the LGBTQ population of interest can assist interventionists in understanding and effectively recruiting participants, discovering appropriate contexts for the delivery of an intervention, and identifying optimal mechanisms of change for that population. Approaching the development of the intervention with a community-involved orientation will assist in the design and implementation of the intervention, and will maximize its reach and impact. Careful consideration of intervention settings, such as online; in homes, schools, places of worship, and the workplace; and community- and clinic-based settings is important for effectively reaching your population. Choosing the optimal mechanism or mechanisms of change—individual, dyadic, small group, community, or structural—will also ensure that your intervention has the broadest impact. Tremendous benefit to the LGBTQ community has been derived from effective approaches to interventions to date. Future efforts should continue to reach out to geographically and culturally isolated segments of the LGBTQ population, to form community partnerships to deliver interventions, and to push for more rigorous evaluation and the development of evidence-based intervention approaches.

References

Abara, W., Coleman, J. D., Fairchild, A., Gaddist, B., and White, J. 2015. A faith-based community partnership to address HIV/AIDS in the Southern United States: Implementation, challenges, and lessons learned. *Journal of Religion and Health* 54(1): 122–33.

Baker, K., McGovern, A., Gruberg, S., and Cray, A. August 9, 2016. *The Medicaid Program and LGBT Communities: Overview and Policy Recommendations.* Retrieved September 12, 2016, from https://www.americanprogress.org/issues/lgbt/report/2016/08/09/142424/the-medicaid-program-and-lgbt-communities-overview-and-policy-recommendations/

Barret, R. L. 1996. Gay fathers in groups. In M. P. Andronico, ed., *Men in Groups: Insights, Interventions, and Psychoeducational Work*, 257–68. Washington, DC: American Psychological Association.

Barron, L. G., and Hebl, M. 2011. Sexual orientation: A protected and unprotected class. In M. A. Paludi, C. J. Paludi, E. R. DeSouza, eds., *Praeger Handbook on Understanding and Preventing Workplace Discrimination*, 2 vols., 251–73. Santa Barbara, CA: Praeger/ABC-CLIO.

Bauermeister, J. A., Meanley, S., Hickok, A., Pingel, E., VanHemert, W., and Loveluck, J. 2014. Sexuality-related work discrimination and its association with the health of sexual minority emerging and young adult men in the Detroit metro area. *Sexuality Research & Social Policy* 11(1): 1–10.

Beatty, J. E., and Kirby, S. L. 2006. Beyond the legal environment: How stigma influences invisible identity groups in the workplace. *Employee Responsibilities and Rights Journal* 18(1): 29–44.

Beyrer, C. 2015. Tailoring biomedical interventions for key populations. *Lancet HIV* 2(1): E8–E9.

Bluespruce, J., Dodge, W. T., Grothaus, L., Wheeler, K., Rebolledo, V., Carey, J. W., and . . . Thompson, R. S. 2000. HIV prevention in primary care: Impact of a clinical intervention. *AIDS Patient Care and Standards* 15(5): 243–53.

Borum, R., and Verhaagen, D. 2006. *Assessing and Managing Violence Risk in Juveniles*. New York: Guilford Press.

Bowen, D. J., Powers, D., and Greenlee, H. 2006. Effects of breast cancer risk counseling for sexual minority women. *Health Care for Women International* 27(1): 45–58.

Bowleg, L., and Bauer, G. 2016. Invited reflection: Quantifying intersectionality. *Psychology of Women Quarterly* 40(3): 337–41.

Bronfenbrenner, U. 1979. *The Ecology of Human Development: Experiments by Nature and Design*. Cambridge, MA: Harvard University Press.

Bronfenbrenner, U. 1986. Ecology of the family as a context for human development: Research perspectives. *Developmental Psychology* 22(6): 723–42.

Bryant, J. 2014. Using respondent-driven sampling with 'hard to reach' marginalised young people: Problems with slow recruitment and small network size. *International Journal of Social Research Methodology: Theory & Practice* 17(6): 599–611.

Chan, C. S. 1995. Issues of sexual identity in an ethnic minority: The case of Chinese American lesbians, gay men, and bisexual people. In A. R. D'Augelli and C. J. Patterson, eds., *Lesbian, Gay, and Bisexual Identities over the Lifespan: Psychological Perspectives*, 87–101. New York: Oxford University Press.

Clark, J. L., Konda, K. A., Silva-Santisteban, A., Peinado, J., Lama, J. R., Kusunoki, L., and . . . Sanchez, J. 2014. Sampling methodologies for epidemiologic surveillance of men who have sex with men and transgender women in Latin America: An empiric comparison of convenience sampling, time-space sampling, and respondent-driven sampling. *AIDS and Behavior* 18(12): 2338–48.

Couper, M. 2000. Review: Web surveys: A review of issues and approaches. *Public Opinion Quarterly* 64(4): 464–94.

Dahlberg, L. L., and Krug, E. G. 2002. Violence: A global health problem. In E. G. Krug et al., eds., *World Report on Violence and Health*. Geneva: World Health Organization.

Doyle-Lindrud, S. 2014. Mobile health technology and the use of health-related mobile applications. *Clinical Journal of Oncology Nursing* 18(6): 634–36.

Eliason, M. J., Dibble, S. L., Gordon, R., and Soliz, G. B. 2012. The last drag: An evaluation of an LGBT-specific smoking intervention. *Journal of Homosexuality* 59(6): 864–78.

Esterberg, K. G. 1996. Gay cultures, gay communities: The social organization of lesbians, gay men, and bisexuals. In K. M. Cohen and R.C. Savin-Williams, eds., *The Lives of Lesbians, Gays, and Bisexuals: Children to Adults*, 377–92. Orlando, FL: Harcourt Brace College Publishers.

Fals-Stewart, W., O'Farrell, T. J., and Lam, W. K. K. 2009. Behavioral couple therapy for gay and lesbian couples with alcohol use disorders. *Journal of Substance Abuse Treatment* 37(4): 379–87.

Family Acceptance Project. http://familyproject.sfsu.edu/

Forrest, J. I., Stevenson, B., Rich, A., Michelow, W., Pai, J., Jollimore, J., and . . . Roth, E. A. 2014. Community mapping and respondent-driven sampling of gay and bisexual men's communities in Vancouver, Canada. *Culture, Health & Sexuality* 16(3): 288–301.

Friends of Project 10: http://friendsofproject10.org/history.html

Frost, D. M., Meyer, I. H., and Schwartz, S. 2016. Social support networks among diverse sexual minority populations. *American Journal of Orthopsychiatry* 86(1): 91–102.

Garnets, L. D., and Kimmel, D. C. 2003. Diversity among lesbians, bisexuals, and gay men. In L. D. Garnets and D. C. Kimmel, eds., *Psychological Perspectives on Lesbian, Gay, and Bisexual Experiences*, 2nd ed. New York: Columbia University Press.

Gibbs, J. J., and Goldbach, J. 2015. Religious conflict, sexual identity, and suicidal behaviors among LGBT young adults. *Archives of Suicide Research* 19(4): 472–88.

Grant, R. M., Anderson, P. L., McMahan, V., Liu, A., Mico, M. M., Hosel, S., et al. 2014. Uptake of pre-exposure prophylaxis, sexual practices, and HIV incidence in men and transgender women who have sex with men: A cohort study. *The Lancet Infectious Diseases* 14: 820–29.

Greenbaum, T. L. 1998. *The Handbook for Focus Group Research*. 2nd ed. Thousand Oaks, CA: Sage Publications.

Grov, C., Rendina, H. J., and Parsons, J. T. 2014. Comparing three cohorts of MSM sampled via sex parties, bars/clubs, and Craigslist.org: Implications for researchers and providers. *AIDS Education and Prevention* 26(4): 362–82.

Hartlieb, K. B., Jacques-Tiura, A. J., Naar-King, S., Ellis, D. A., Catherine Jen, K., and Marshall, S. 2015. Recruitment strategies and the retention of obese urban racial/ethnic minority adolescents in clinical trials: The FIT Families Project, Michigan, 2010–2014. *Preventing Chronic Disease: Public Health Research, Practice, and Policy* 12.

Hash, K. M., and Rogers, A. 2013. Clinical practice with older LGBT clients: Overcoming lifelong stigma through strength and resilience. *Clinical Social Work Journal* 41(3): 249–57.

Hirshfield, S., Grov, C., Parsons, J. T., Anderson, I., and Chiasson, M. A. 2015. Social media use and HIV transmission risk behavior among ethnically diverse HIV-positive gay men: Results of an online study in three U.S. States. *Archives of Sexual Behavior* 44(7): 1969–78.

HIV/AIDS Prevention Research Synthesis Project (Centers for Disease Control and Prevention). Updated November–December 2019. *Compendium of Evidence-Based Interventions and Best Practices for HIV Prevention*. https:www.cdc.gov/hiv/research/interventionresearch/compendium/index.html.

Holmes, S. E., and Cahill, S. 2004. School experiences of gay, lesbian, bisexual and transgender youth. *Journal of Gay & Lesbian Issues in Education* 1(3): 53–66.

Human Rights Campaign, http://www.hrc.org/resources/diversity-training-on-sexual-orientation-and-gender-identity-issues, retrieved April 20, 2016

Hunt, C. M., Davidson, M. J., Fielden, S. L., and Hoel, H. 2010. Reviewing sexual harassment in the workplace—An intervention model. *Personnel Review* 39(5): 655–73.

Institute of Medicine. 2011. *The Health of Lesbian, Gay, Bisexual, and Transgender People: Building a Foundation for Better Understanding*. Washington, DC: National Academies Press.

Jeffries, W. I. 2011. The number of recent sex partners among bisexual men in the United States. *Perspectives on Sexual and Reproductive Health* 43(3): 151–57.

Kamen, C., McMahon, J. M., Heckler, C., Heffner, K., Morrow, G. R., Mustian, K. and Bowen, D. 2016. Recruitment and retention of lesbian, gay, bisexual, and transgender cancer survivors and their caregivers to a randomized behavioral intervention trial: Feasibility and lessons learned. Unpublished manuscript.

Kazyak, E. 2012. Midwest or lesbian? Gender, rurality, and sexuality. *Gender & Society* 26(6): 825–48

Kimmel, D. C., Rose, T., and David, S. 2006. *Lesbian, Gay, Bisexual, and Transgender Aging: Research and Clinical Perspectives*. New York: Columbia University Press.

Kitts, R. L. 2010. Barriers to optimal care between physicians and lesbian, gay, bisexual, transgender, and questioning adolescent patients. *Journal of Homosexuality* 57(6): 730–47.

Kirby, T., and Thornber-Dunwell, M. 2014. Phone apps could help promote sexual health in MSM. *Lancet* 384(9952): 1415.

Ko, N., Lee, H., Hung, C., Chang, J., Lee, N., Chang, C., and . . . Ko, W. (2009). Effects of structural intervention on increasing condom availability and reducing risky sexual behaviours in gay bathhouse attendees. *AIDS Care* 21(12): 1499–1507.

Lambda Legal 2010. When health care isn't caring: Lambda Legal's survey on discrimination against LGBT people and people living with HIV. Available at: http://data.lambdalegal.org/publications/downloads/whcicreport_when-health-care-isnt-caring.pdf. Accessed January 2, 2017

Lambda Legal. 2017. *Employment: Demanding Workplace Equality*: http://www.lambdalegal.org/issues/employment-and-rights-in-the-workplace.

Macapagal, K., Bhatia, R., and Greene, G. J. 2016. Differences in healthcare access, use, and experiences within a community sample of racially diverse lesbian, gay, bisexual, transgender, and questioning emerging adults. *LGBT Health* 3(6): 434–42.

Magnus, M., Kuo, I., Shelley, K., Rawls, A., Peterson, J., Montanez, L., and . . . Greenberg, A. E. 2009. Risk factors driving the emergence of a generalized heterosexual HIV epidemic in Washington, District of Columbia, networks at risk. *AIDS* 23(10): 1277–84.

Martinez, O., Wu, E., Levine, E. C., Muñoz-Laboy, M., Fernandez, M. I., Bass, S. B., and . . . Rhodes, S. D. 2016. Integration of social, cultural, and biomedical strategies into an existing couple-based behavioral HIV/STI prevention intervention: Voices of Latino male couples. *Plos ONE* 11(3).

Martinez, O., Wu, E., Shultz, A. Z., Capote, J., Rios, J. L., Sandfort, T., and . . . Rhodes, S. D. 2014. Still a hard-to-reach population? Using social media to recruit Latino gay couples for an HIV intervention adaptation study. *Journal of Medical Internet Research* 16(4): 1–14.

Meyer, I. H., and Bayer, R. 2013. School-based gay-affirmative interventions: First amendment and ethical concerns. *American Journal of Public Health* 103(10): 1764–71.

Molock, S., Zea, M. C., Reisen, C. A., and Poppen, P.J. Pilot to increase HIV testing among African American youth in black churches. Unpublished manuscript.

Mustanski, B., Greene, G. J., Ryan, D., and Whitton, S. W. 2015. Feasibility, acceptability, and initial efficacy of an online sexual health promotion program for LGBT youth: The Queer Sex Ed intervention. *Journal of Sex Research* 52(2): 220–30.

Montgomery, C. M., Watts, C., and Pool, R. 2012. HIV and dyadic intervention: An interdependence and communal coping analysis. *PLoS One* 7(7)

Mutchler, M. G., McKay, T., McDavitt, B., and Gordon, K. K. 2013. Using peer ethnography to address health disparities among young urban Black and Latino men who have sex with men. *American Journal of Public Health* 103(5): 849–52.

Nadal, K. Y. 2011. Responding to racial, gender, and sexual orientation micro-aggressions in the workplace. In M. A. Paludi, C. J. Paludi, and E. R. DeSouza, eds., *Praeger Handbook on Understanding and Preventing Workplace Discrimination*, 23–32. Santa Barbara, CA: Praeger/ABC-CLIO.

Nation, R. A. 2016. HIV and Black mistrust of the healthcare system and medical research: Plenary presentation at the GLMA Health Professionals Advancing LGBT Health Conference, St. Louis.

Ng, H. H. 2016. Intersectionality and shared decision making in LGBTQ health. *LGBT Health* 3(5): 325–26.

Northridge, M. E., McGrath, B. P., and Krueger, S. Q. 2007. Using community-based participatory research to understand and eliminate social disparities in health for lesbian, gay, bisexual, and transgender populations. In I. H. Meyer and M. E. Northridge, eds., *The Health of Sexual Minorities: Public Health Perspectives on Lesbian, Gay, Bisexual, and Transgender Populations*, 455–70. New York: Springer Science and Business Media.

Pantalone, D. W., Bimbi, D. S., Holder, C. A., Golub, S. A., and Parsons, J. T. 2010. Consistency and change in club drug use by sexual minority men in New York City, 2002 to 2007. *American Journal of Public Health* 100(10): 1892–95.

Poteat, V. P., Scheer, J. R., Marx, R. A., Calzo, J. P., and Yoshikawa, H. 2015. Gay-Straight Alliances vary on dimensions of youth socializing and advocacy: Factors accounting for individual and setting-level differences. *American Journal of Community Psychology* 55(3–4): 422–32.

Przybyla, S. M. 2010. Examining correlates of serostatus disclosure and sexual transmission risk behaviors among people living with HIV in North Carolina. *Dissertation Abstracts International* 70: 4121.

Quintanilla, M. 1989. Haven for Gay Teens: Education: Some people call Project 10 a bad idea, but the counseling program gives some homosexual students in L.A. the courage to stay in school. *Los Angeles Times,* December 7, 1989. Retrieved September 12, 2016, from http://articles.latimes.com/1989-12-07/news/vw-404_1_gay-teens

Reitman, D. S., Austin, B., Belkind, U., Chaffee, T., Hoffman, N. D., Moore, E., and . . . Ryan, C. 2013. Recommendations for promoting the health and well-being of lesbian, gay, bisexual, and transgender adolescents: A position paper of the society for adolescent health and medicine. *Journal of Adolescent Health* 52(4): 506–10.

Rizer, A. M., Mauery, D. R., Haynes, S. G., Couser, B., and Gruman, C. 2015. Challenges in intervention research for lesbian and bisexual women. *LGBT Health* 2(2): 105–12.

Rosenthal, L. (2016). Incorporating intersectionality into psychology: An opportunity to promote social justice and equity. *American Psychologist* 71(6): 474–85.

Russell, S. T., Muraco, A., Subramaniam, A., and Laub, C. 2009. Youth empowerment and high school gay-straight alliances. *Youth Adolescence* 38(7): 891–903.

Ryan, C., and Chen-Hayes, S. F. 2013. Educating and empowering families of lesbian, gay, bisexual, transgender, and questioning students. In E. S. Fisher, K. Komosa-Hawkins, E. S. Fisher, and K. Komosa-Hawkins, eds., *Creating Safe and Supportive Learning Environments: A Guide for Working with Lesbian, Gay, Bisexual, Transgender, and Questioning Youth and Families*, 209–29. New York: Routledge/Taylor & Francis.

Ryan, C., Huebner, D., Diaz, R., and Sanchez, J. 2009. Family rejection as a predictor of negative health outcomes in White and Latino lesbian, gay, and bisexual young adults. *Pediatrics* 123: 346–52.

Ryan, C., Russell, S. T., Huebner, D., Diaz, R., and Sanchez, J. 2010. Family acceptance in adolescence and the health of LGBT young adults. *Journal of Child and Adolescent Psychiatric Nursing* 23(4): 205–13.

Schoenberg, N. E., Bundy, H. E., Bispo, J. B., Studts, C. R., Shelton, B. J., and Fields, N. 2015. A rural Appalachian faith-placed smoking cessation intervention. *Journal of Religion and Health* 54(2): 598–611.

Skerrett, D. M., and Mars, M. 2014. Addressing the social determinants of suicidal behaviors and poor mental health in LGBTI populations in Australia. *LGBT Health* 1(3): 212–17.

Smalley, K. B., Warren, J. C., and Barefoot, K. N. 2016. Differences in health risk behaviors across understudied LGBT subgroups. *Health Psychology* 35(2): 103–14.

Sun, C. J., García, M., Mann, L., Alonzo, J., Eng, E., and Rhodes, S. D. 2015. Latino sexual and gender identity minorities promoting sexual health within their social networks: Process evaluation findings from a lay health advisor intervention. *Health Promotion Practice* 16(3): 329–37.

Szabo, S. M., Whitlatch, C. J., Orsulic-Jeras, S., and Johnson, J. D. 2016. Recruitment challenges and strategies: Lessons learned from an early-stage dyadic intervention (innovative practice). *Dementia* 17(5): 621–26.

Teo, A. R., Andrea, S. B., Sakakibara, R., Motohara, S., Matthieu, M. M., and Fetters, M. D. 2016. Brief gatekeeper training for suicide prevention in an ethnic minority population: A controlled intervention. *BMC Psychiatry* 16, article 11.

Thompson, S., Forssell, S., and Wunder, K. 2008. Increasing PLWH involvement in HIV planning and advocacy activities in local U.S. communities through training and follow-up. Poster presentation at the International AIDS Conference, Mexico City, Mexico.

Thurston, I. B., Bogart, L. M., Wachman, M., Closson, E. F., Skeer, M. R., and Mimiaga, M. J. 2014. Adaptation of an HIV medication adherence intervention for adolescents and young adults. *Cognitive and Behavioral Practice* 21(2): 191–205.

Timmons, S. M. 2015. Review and evaluation of faith-based weight management interventions that target African American women. *Journal of Religion and Health* 54(2): 798–809.

Tourangeau, R., Edwards, B., Johnson, T. P., Wolter, K. M., and Bates, N. 2014. *Hard-to-survey Populations*. New York: Cambridge University Press.

US Department of Health and Human Services. 2015. *Framework: The Vision, Mission and Goals of* Healthy People 2020. Retrieved from http://www.healthypeople.gov/sites/default/files/HP2020Framework.pdf.

Walker, J. J., and Longmire-Avital, B. 2013. The impact of religious faith and internalized homonegativity on resiliency for black lesbian, gay, and bisexual emerging adults. *Developmental Psychology* 49(9): 1723–31.

Wallerstein, N. B., and Duran, B. 2006. Using community-based participatory research to address health disparities. *Health Promotion Practice* 7(3): 312–23.

Walls, N. E., and Wisneski, H. 2011. Evaluation of smoking cessation classes for the lesbian, gay, bisexual, and transgender community. *Journal of Social Service Research* 37(1): 99–111.

Wanigaratne, S., Billington, A., and Williams, M. 1997. Initiating and maintaining safer sex: Evaluation of group work with gay men. In J. Catalán, L. Sherr, and B. Hedge, eds., *The Impact of AIDS: Psychological and Social Aspects of HIV Infection*, 27–41. Amsterdam: Harwood Academic Publishers.

Wolff, J. R., Himes, H. L., Soares, S. D., and Miller Kwon, E. 2016. Sexual minority students in non-affirming religious higher education: Mental health, outness, and identity. *Psychology of Sexual Orientation and Gender Diversity* 3(2): 201–12.

Zule, W. A., Bobashev, G. V., Wechsberg, W. M., Costenbader, E. C., and Coomes, C. M. 2009. Behaviorally bisexual men and their risk behaviors with men and women. *Journal of Urban Health* 86(S1): 48–62.

THIRTEEN

Program Development Considerations for LGBTQ Health Interventions

José A. Bauermeister, Ryan C. Tingler, and Gary W. Harper

HEALTH PROMOTION programs and interventions are most effective when they are informed by a systematic program-planning process (McKenzie 2013). As a process, program planning can help identify and address the socioecological correlates affecting the health and well-being of LGBTQ people and their communities. Program planners sometimes distinguish between "interventions" and "programs." *Interventions* refer to one or more planned activities that are developed and delivered during a specified period with the intent of improving health, whereas *programs* may be broader than an intervention and include several different interventions. We use these terms interchangeably in this chapter to describe planned activities that are designed and delivered based on health behavior theories. This chapter provides a synopsis of several program-planning considerations when developing or adapting interventions and programs for LGBTQ populations.

Program-planning frameworks (e.g., Intervention Mapping, RE-AIM, PRECEDE-PROCEED) are employed by public health practitioners to design new programs or interventions, or to adapt existing evidence-based programs for new populations or modes of delivery (Bartholomew, Parcel, Kok, and Gottlieb 2001; Glasgow 2002; Green and Kreuter

2005). These frameworks often detail the various steps that should be taken when developing, implementing, and evaluating health promotion programs. Although each planning framework may place different emphasis on the steps to be taken during the planning process, they all share the same purpose: to create health promotion programs that are responsive to the needs of diverse communities using theoretically informed strategies and that can be delivered and evaluated in a culturally responsive manner. Apart from HIV/STI prevention and care interventions designed for sexual and gender minority populations, there are a limited number of interventions developed or adapted specifically to address LGBTQ health issues (Institute of Medicine 2011). Consequently, throughout this chapter we emphasize the value and importance of participatory planning processes when seeking to develop health programs for LGBTQ populations and communities.

Participatory Approaches to Program Development

Participatory action research (PAR) is an interactive, reflective process that seeks to continually identify and prioritize the problems in a community and create and implement interventions in a participatory way (MacQueen et al. 2001). PAR methods are often used during the program-planning process given their potential to engage multiple stakeholders within a community; to benefit from the perspective, expertise, and experience from communities affected by the issue; and to increase buy-in during the development and implementation process. For example, Ryan and colleagues (2012) developed the Family Acceptance Project using a PAR process to develop, implement, evaluate, and disseminate a program focused on preventing and reducing the social, physical, and mental health risks affecting LGBTQ children and youth. Using in-depth interviews and surveys, Ryan et al. (2012) have incorporated feedback from LGBTQ youth, families, and health providers (e.g., mental health practitioners, teachers, social workers, and advocates) to successfully execute the project. The collective input from diverse constituents has led to the development of family-based strategies focused on decreasing familial rejection and increasing health promotive resources among LGBTQ youth belonging to ethnically and religiously diverse families in the United States.

Community-based participatory research (CBPR) is the most popular PAR approach used in public health. CBPR seeks to build on participatory action research and empowerment values (Israel, Lantz, McGranaghan, Kerr, and Guzman 2005; Israel, Schulz, Parker, and Becker, 1998; Israel et al. 2003) by challenging the notion of "researcher-as-expert" and centering and valuing community practice expertise and lived experience. Participatory research approaches build upon many principles, including co-learning, power-sharing, and building community capacity; focus on the local relevance of health problems; and involve a cyclical and iterative process (Meredith Minkler and Wallerstein 2003). Rather than relying on a deficit model, CBPR approaches often draw from communities' assets and resources to identify priorities, decision-making strategies, and implementation approaches (Eng and Blanchard, 1997; McKnight and Kretzmann, 1996). These efforts help to reinforce community ownership of health promotion priorities and strategies, and can promote program acceptability and adoption, as well as long-term sustainability. Bryant, Damarin, and Marshall (2014) used a CBPR approach when developing Project Muse, a tobacco-control project for LGBTQ individuals in Atlanta. The team credits the use of participatory approaches for the creation of a process that supported the institutionalization and sustainability of a community partnership. By having the research team, community advisory board, members of Atlanta's Black gay community, and former smokers contribute to the project, the research team was able to obtain deeper insights on how to reduce LGBTQ tobacco use through collaborative partnerships.

Although PAR definitions and approaches vary in the program planning literature, the variability in PAR's operationalization is attributable to communities' level of involvement during the identification and prioritization of the health problem, and their subsequent participation in the program's design, implementation, and evaluation. Arnstein's (1969) ladder of citizen participation helps to illustrate the variability in participation and power between researchers, program planners, and community members, representing varying degrees of power held by community members during the intervention.

The first two rungs (manipulation and therapy) of Arnstein's ladder are described as nonparticipation processes whereby external stakeholders (e.g., public health departments, policymakers, researchers) assume that community members are unaware of the issues affecting their community and therefore must be "educated" without any say in the intervention process. The third (informing) and fourth (consultation) rungs allow community members to hear and have a voice, but they have no power to ensure that their voice has influence. At the fifth rung (placation), community members are perceived as advisors, yet the external stakeholders retain the control of the decision-making process. Arnstein's last three rungs are often described as "true participation" and posited to be most effective given that community members have decision-making power and a voice in the allocation of resources and strategies. Within the sixth rung (participation), community members can negotiate and have shared decision-making responsibility and accountability. At the seventh rung (delegated power) and eighth rung (citizen control), community members account for most of the power in the decision-making process.

The imagery proposed by Arnstein's ladder is helpful, as it emphasizes the importance of monitoring power dynamics throughout the life of a program (Harper, Contreras, Bangi, and Pedraza 2003; Zimmerman 2000). For instance, ensuring that community participation is as active in later stages (e.g., helping analyze the data during program evaluation) as it was during the formative stages of the planning process (e.g., recruitment) may reduce feelings of being used or tokenized. Similarly, if a program is evaluated as efficacious, new strategies (e.g., trainer of trainers) may be required to increase a community's involvement during the scale-up and sustainability phases. For the remainder of this chapter, we focus on strategies and processes that seek to be conscious of community participation and empowerment.

Stakeholders' Involvement in the Development of an HIV Prevention Intervention for Young Black Gay and Bisexual Men in Chicago

Gary W. Harper

A Youth Action Board (YAB) facilitated the development of an HIV prevention intervention as part of a community-based participatory research project. YAB members were young Black gay/bisexual men ages 19–24 with experience working in a variety of roles throughout the LGBTQ community. The YAB was instrumental in the development of the intervention, including co-analyzing data from prior studies, naming the intervention, identifying topics for the intervention, developing intervention activities, and assisting in participant recruitment. The YAB assisted in tailoring materials used in the intervention to be culturally and developmentally appropriate to young gay and bisexual men.

YAB members were trained in a critical consciousness-coaching technique and subsequently involved in intervention delivery sessions as cofacilitators. On the basis of their participation in the intervention, the YAB began to apply critical consciousness concepts to their daily lives and professional development. Since their initial involvement in the project, several YAB members have enrolled in institutions of higher learning, while others have advanced in their work environments. These findings highlight the value that community-based participatory research approaches can have in building the strengths and skill sets of community members.

LGBTQ Interventions Require Partnerships

Beyond involvement of community members, partnerships often include officials from public health departments, faith-based leaders, community advocates, and/or staff from community-based organizations. Their involvement is often recommended, as they can help to promote the development and implementation of multisectoral and community-driven solutions. Further, in pooling their resources and expertise, these partnerships may be better equipped to recognize multilevel barriers to optimal prevention and care, and to develop structural and community interventions aimed at reducing systemic deficiencies. Seelman and colleagues (2016) demonstrated the importance of community partnerships when conducting their study assessing interventions for healthy aging among mature Black lesbians. By collaborating with networks of Black LGBTQ organizations and key gatekeepers in the region to reach their population, the research team was able to recruit 100 mature Black lesbians to engage in the study and to offer key recommendations for interventions promoting healthy aging in their community.

Several frameworks have been developed to provide guidance in the formation and maintenance of collaborative partnerships. The Interactive and Contextual Model of Collaboration (Suarez-Balcazar, Harper, and Lewis 2005) is unique in that it articulates a range of issues and factors to address in the process of developing and sustaining collaborations, and elaborates specific principles and values that influence the process of the relationship trajectory while also addressing the potential challenges and threats to the collaboration. The phases of the Interactive and Contextual Model of Collaboration comprise (1) gaining entry into the community, (2) developing and sustaining a mutual collaboration (developing trust and mutual respect, establishing adequate communication, respecting human diversity, establishing a culture of learning, respecting the culture of the setting and the community, and developing an action agenda), and (3) recognizing the benefits and outcomes of partnership work. The model also includes the potential challenges that might threaten the partnership, such as resource inequality and time commitment.

Summary. Collaborative partnerships between researchers and community stakeholders can help create LGBTQ health interventions that are relevant and responsive to the community's needs. We highlight some best practices to ensure active community involvement based on lessons learned from the Project VIDA Case Study (Harper et al. 2004) below.

Social Diagnosis in Intervention Planning

Community-engaged processes recognize that communities should have the capacity to advocate for health promotion conditions in order to materialize and control the psychosocial and biological factors influencing

Collaborative Partnership Development and Maintenance: Project VIDA

A collaborative partnership between a Latino-focused community-based organization and a team of university-based evaluators was formed to evaluate HIV prevention interventions for Mexican American female adolescents and gay/bisexual/questioning Latino male adolescents. In creating and enhancing a reciprocal and mutually beneficial relationship, the partnership overcame challenges during the formation and maintenance of their collaborative partnership. The best practices for community collaboration were divided into three domains (Building Relationships; Building on Existing Strengths; and Building a Sense of Commitment to the Project) and summarized below.

Building Relationships
1. Invest time in sharing information about work-related constraints, demands, and dynamics;
2. Clearly define each research/evaluation team member's roles and responsibilities;
3. Learn about unique community and agency cultures by participating in activities and events;
4. Share belief and value systems about working with diverse populations; and
5. Recognize, respect, and participate in agency rituals and traditions to foster trust and comfort.

Building on Existing Strengths
1. Create strategies for decreasing power differentials (e.g., conduct meetings at the agency, alternate facilitators);
2. Work with supervisory staff to decrease or shift staff members' competing responsibilities;
3. Conduct educational sessions to explain the purpose and results of the research/evaluation project;
4. Assess the necessary skills and resources required for the completion of research/evaluation activities; and
5. Provide resources, support, and training to increase and maintain competencies.

Building a Sense of Commitment to the Project
1. Create efficient methods to communicate information within the team and with agency staff;
2. Create a research/evaluation plan with recognizable benefits that includes short- and long-term goals;

3. Elicit and incorporate input from all team members throughout the collaboration;
4. Provide individualized training and support to new members who join the team; and
5. Provide a visual timeline of accomplishments to acknowledge members' contributions.

their health through coordinated and equitable participation. Once a partnership has been established, it is common to carry out a needs assessment to understand the problem and its root causes, as well as to gauge the resources and assets available within the community. Consistent with the participatory approach of this chapter, we encourage the use of social diagnosis methods during intervention planning rather than traditional, top-down nonparticipatory needs-assessment methods.

The Action-Oriented Community Diagnosis method (Eng and Blanchard 1997) is a popular community-driven social diagnosis approach. This participatory approach examines the psychosocial conditions affecting health behaviors and outcomes and systematically proposes steps to maximize multisectoral participation, refine the constituents' needs and priorities, and increase communities' collective competence to develop potential solutions. This process often relies on iterative review of data and community participation. Data collection methods described earlier in this book (see chapter **), whether they be primary and/or secondary in nature, can be used during the social diagnosis phase. These efforts should reflect the spirit of multisector partnerships and collaborations, and precede the development or adaptation of intervention strategies and materials to ensure that they are reflective of the focus populations. Below, we outline several sources of data that facilitate this process.

Existing Data

Prior to any new data collection, program planners often recommend the thorough review of the literature and accessing existing data in the community. Existing data may include available datasets (e.g., census and health department datasets), prior needs assessments, findings from evaluations of interventions/policies previously implemented in the community, and reports from local advocacy groups and/or government planning groups. Researchers will often use behavioral data to inform interventions. For example, building on the existing literature documenting the role of minority stress in the health outcomes of gay and bisexual men, Pachankis and colleagues (2015) adapted the Unified Protocol intervention, focusing on stigma-based coping as a strategy to improve depression, anxiety, and co-occurring health risks of young adult gay and bisexual men.

The review of risk indicators should receive attention equal to the resources and assets in the community. Further, care should be taken when relying on existing data. Specifically, it is important to understand the sources of these data (e.g., who were the stakeholders consulted during the original data collection?) and to note whether specific community sectors were excluded in prior efforts. Understanding gaps in the available evidence can help contextualize these findings, as well as help program planners decide whether the social diagnosis might benefit from primary data collection.

Formative Data

Primary data collection (e.g., preliminary data, pilot data) might be necessary if the program planning group identifies gaps within the existing data, desires the community's opinions and enthusiasm for intervention strategies being considered, and/or wishes to pilot-test the evaluation assessments to be used during the program implementation phase.

The use of survey methods to understand individuals' perceptions, experiences, and behaviors may be useful to inform intervention strategies and mechanisms of change. Surveys (see chapter 12) may also be helpful to understand the prevalence of social, environmental, and interpersonal characteristics, as well as to rank and/or prioritize elements under consideration as potential intervention strategies. In order to understand the perceived importance of five different health issues (i.e.,

HIV/STDs, drugs and alcohol, body image, mental health, and smoking) for gay and bisexual men, Grov and colleagues (2012) used brief, anonymous surveys of men in gay bars/clubs and bathhouses in New York City. Using a brief survey (3–5 minutes) allowed the research team to gather valuable data and prioritize the importance of these health issues among community members. This efficient and effective method of data collection provided researchers with data to inform comprehensive approaches to health education and outreach for gay and bisexual men in urban settings (Grov 2012).

Focus Groups and In-Depth Interviews

Focus groups and in-depth interviews may be useful qualitative strategies to acquire additional information necessary during the formative phase of the intervention planning process. Like their use in basic public health research (see chapter 6), questions may seek to understand how determinants of interest influence individual and community behaviors. However, focus groups and in-depth interviews may also be well suited to assess vital information linked to the potential success and feasibility of the intervention. For example, a program planner may wish to assess stakeholders' and collaborators' enthusiasm for the proposed intervention and/or brainstorm with them how to achieve buy-in, as well as to examine how participants describe the problems faced in their communities and brainstorm ideas on how to solve these problems within their community. Carter and colleagues (2012) used focus groups and in-depth interviews during the initial stages of their research study aiming to increase access to cervical screening for lesbian and bisexual women. By using this approach to gather data from participants, the facilitators were able to generate qualitative content regarding the lack of cervical screenings for lesbian and bisexual women. This allowed practitioners to understand the problems that lesbian and bisexual women face when seeking cervical screenings.

Power Mapping

Power mapping is a qualitative tool often used in program planning to identify who is involved in community decision-making (e.g., community advocates, nonprofit organizations, corporations, government institutions, funders, political and religious leaders) and the relationships and networks between these different groups (Brown 2003; McKnight and Kretzmann 1996). Power-mapping data may be useful to leverage political will, develop persuasive campaigns that increase the acceptability of your intervention, and/or plan for resistance from different sectors. Power-mapping data may also facilitate the selection of settings (e.g., home, clubs, clinics, faith-based agencies) and channels (e.g., face-to-face, peer leaders, online) through which to deliver intervention content. Below, we present an example on how mixed-methods data were used as part of iterative, community-based discussions that relied on formative data and power-mapping strategies to inform the selection and design of a health program for sexual and gender minorities (Bauermeister et al. 2017).

Ensuring Community Input in the Development of Structural Interventions for Young Queer Men and Transgender Women

A Case Study from the Michigan Forward in Enhancing Research and Community Equity (MFierce)

A coalition (Michigan Forward in Enhancing Research and Community Equity, or MFierce) comprising youth advisors, health department officials, community organizations, and university researchers was created in August 2014. MFierce uses a community-based participatory research approach to engage researchers and community partners through shared decision-making. This community engagement approach offered an alternative to traditional research by challenging the notion of "researcher-as-expert" and centering community expertise and lived experience. We employed a three-round process to synthesize ideas that could inform our community-level intervention.

In Round 1 (Idea Generation), we held eight community dialogues in which participants wrote down goals that could improve the sexual health of sexual minority men and gender minority women in southeast Michigan. Participants shared the goals with the larger group and placed their notes at the front of the room. As a group, participants then devised strategies that the coalition might consider implementing. The goals were often broad and vague yet offered concrete ideas for the coalition to think about ways to move forward. Each community dialogue ended with a debriefing session and time allotted to complete the evaluation. Once the eight dialogues were completed, the entire coalition held a retreat to discuss and prioritize the ideas that had been generated. Coalition members identified their top choices for project directions based on considerations of the feasibility, acceptability, and desirability of each idea. This process resulted in a list of twelve potential intervention areas.

In Round 2 (Idea Refinement), we held three community dialogues focused on activities that could advance the intervention area. At each dialogue, participants were given three stickers—one red, one yellow, and one green—with their top three choices (green = first choice; red = third choice). The intervention areas that received the most votes (three to four areas out of twelve) were announced. Participants then split up into three or four groups, and each group was given nearly an hour to create their own design for an intervention in their area. The facilitators provided each group with a "project mapping" worksheet that served as a guide. The worksheet included boxes in which participants detailed what the project would require in terms of resources, materials, and personnel, the primary activities that composed the project, and the anticipated impact upon HIV/STI rates among YGB-MTW in southeast Michigan. Each group presented their idea at the end and had the opportunity to field questions. Using these project maps, coalition members discussed and sketched further details for each proposal, consolidating several of the proposal ideas where overlaps occurred. This led to the synthesis of seven proposal ideas.

In Round 3 (Prioritization), we held a single culminating event that the coalition dubbed "The Summit." The coalition presented seven final ideas to community members using a roundtable (e.g., speed dating) format. Summit participants were assigned to a group (that was presented on their nametag upon entry), and their group would spend 15 minutes at each of the tables, gradually making their way around over a two-hour period. At each roundtable session, the coalition members representing the table would introduce their proposal, communicate key points regarding the significance and impact of the work, and elucidate five specific activities to be imple-

(continued)

mented in service of the project. Participants then had the opportunity to voice concerns or questions. After visiting all seven tables, attendees were treated to lunch and asked to vote on the proposal they perceived to have the greatest impact, feasibility, and need. These questionnaires were then collected and used to modify each proposal in preparation for the Coalition's final selection of intervention strategies to be designed and implemented.

After the community dialogues had concluded, MFierce held several all-coalition, in-person meetings to decide which strategies to formally adopt based on the data and information from this iterative process. Two proposals were selected and moved forward: a Health Access Initiative (HAI) and an Advocacy Collective (AC). HAI seeks to offer healthcare providers across southeast Michigan with cultural humility training focused on young sexual and gender minority youth, whereas the AC is a training program for young sexual and gender minority youth to learn consulting and advocacy roles. Both projects are currently being implemented and evaluated in southeast Michigan.

Photovoice is an increasingly popular form of participant observation that also helps to persuade constituents about a community's needs and experiences. Photovoice encourages people, as participant-photographers, to identify, represent, and enact social change in their community through photographs (Wang and Burris 1997; Wang, Yi, Tao, and Carovano 1998). Photovoice provides cameras to participant-photographers and encourages them to actively record and evidence their communities' strengths and weaknesses in order to promote social change (Wang, Yi, Tao, and Carovano 1998). This process can be empowering to participants, as it provides a process by which they may photograph their social realities and find meaning in them (Wang and Burris 1997). Most importantly, the Photovoice process heightens participants' understanding of their realities and allows the participant-photographers to share their experiences with other members of the community, including other participants, community leaders, policymakers, and stakeholders.

Summary. A comprehensive needs assessment can be participatory in nature and rely on multiple sources (e.g., surveys, interviews, photos), providing multiple perspectives to optimize diversity and inclusion.

Photolove

Employing Photovoice to Understand Young Gay and Bisexual Men's Dating Behaviors

Rachael Strecher and José A. Bauermeister

Love and relationships are salient topics in sex education, yet we're often challenged to put the concept of love into words. As a MPH student at the University of Michigan, Rachael Strecher developed a Photovoice project ("Photolove") focused on young gay and bisexual men's sexual and partner-seeking behaviors. Photolove gave study participants an opportunity to explain their perspectives on love, using both words and images. If they met the study requirements (between the ages of 18 and 24, and identifying as gay, bisexual, queer, or questioning), they chose whether they wanted to create a collage or take photographs that represented their conception of romantic love. If they chose the photography option, we sent them a disposable camera and a prepaid and addressed envelope in which to return it. If they created a collage, they could bring it to the in-depth interview or email it to us in advance. Once they sent us the creative portion of the project, we scheduled a one-hour in-depth interview where participants shared how feelings of love, friendship, and desire align with their sexual health and dating behaviors. We transcribed, coded, and analyzed these texts and imagery.

So what is love according to the young men we interviewed? As you might imagine, love represented an amalgam of experiences. To one participant, whose collage showed a field filled with hundreds of flowers, with one person bringing flowers to another, love manifested itself as romance. To another participant, a recent immigrant from Mexico, love was acceptance of his sexuality—by himself and by others. For other men, love took on a new future that included marriage, children, and growing old together given advances in LGBTQ rights (fig. 13.1).

Is a picture worth more than a thousand words? In our case, the answer was yes. This methodology helped us enrich our qualitative formative work and helped us identify themes not often included in comprehensive sex education for sexual minority men. Photovoice offered young men an opportunity to describe and share complex components of their sexuality and lives through a creative, participatory

(continued)

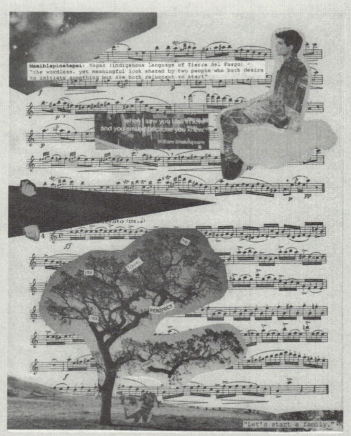

Figure 13.1. Collage created by a Photolove participant to represent the development of a relationship over time. Used with permission.

process. We have used their creations to inform the design and development of a comprehensive sex education intervention for single, same sex–attracted young men. This intervention is currently being pilot-tested for feasibility and preliminary efficacy.

Furthermore, the analysis of needs-assessment data can be used to garner input from stakeholders and relevant members of the LGBTQ population in order to identify the most suitable intervention strategies (i.e., as defined by their feasibility, priority, and effectiveness) or to exclude potential approaches with limited support and/or enthusiasm.

Intervention Development

LGBTQ interventions are often designed using intervention activities or programmatic elements found to be acceptable and/or efficacious in other populations. As a result, it is often useful to review existing program materials and protocols and verify whether they might be adapted for the LGBTQ population of interest. Using needs-assessment data and/or evaluation data from an existing intervention, program planners can design components that foresee the maximum feasible uptake and participation from the intended population. For example, Senreich (2010) examined whether sexual minorities who participated in a LGBTQ specialized treatment had improved outcomes (e.g., abstinence) when compared with peers in a traditional (e.g., heterosexual) treatment program. Findings suggested that programs with LGBTQ program components were more favorable than traditional programs, underscoring the need to build programs that are relevant and specific to the intended population. In this section of the chapter, we highlight key considerations when culturally tailoring or culturally adapting interventions to LGBTQ populations.

Developing an Intervention

As an intervention is designed, its goals must align with the appropriate mechanism of change and mode of delivery, have theoretically supported intervention activities, and be reflective of the populations' needs (see chapter 12). There is often a temptation to use "pre-packaged" interventions since they have already developed intervention manuals, guides, and implementation materials. Before using a pre-packaged intervention, however, it is important to first determine whether the intended outcomes of the intervention match the needs and wants of the community. Consistent with the social diagnosis process described earlier in the chapter, just because an existing program focuses generally on some aspect of LGBTQ health does not mean that it is appropriate for or desired by your specific community.

Program planners may use the needs-assessment data (e.g., existing data, formative data) collected during the social diagnosis phase to determine whether the needs of the community are best served by building a new intervention or program, whether a pre-packaged intervention is suitable for implementation (particularly if it can leverage existing services or resources in the community), and/or whether pre-packaged and existing programs can supplement each other (as opposed to adapting and implementing a whole new intervention). As a note of caution, supplementation of existing programs may require collaborative engagement with other public health entities and could involve programmatic challenges, particularly if agencies do not wish to relinquish control over the design of their pre-packaged interventions (Dworkin, Pinto, Hunter, Rapkin, and Remien 2008). Assuming an agreement can be reached, the program planning team can now begin to design the intervention content or adapt a pre-packaged intervention.

The following are useful steps to begin the design of an intervention or program (for an in-depth description of the intervention development process, see Bartholomew et al. 2001). It is helpful to construct an advisory board that is constituted from members of the focal population that you want to serve. It also may be helpful to construct a second advisory board that includes members from the communities/agencies/organizations that will eventually be delivering your intervention to the focal population. The advisory board(s) can help analyze the formative work collected during the social diagnosis phase and provide insights into how different community groups might conceptualize and understand the focal behaviors to be addressed in the intervention, as well as their psychosocial determinants. Once these data have been analyzed and discussed with appropriate advisory boards, the program planners should work collaboratively with the advisory boards to create a conceptual model for the intervention based on health behavior change theory. Once a conceptual model is agreed upon, program planners can begin to outline intervention activities and strategies that align with the theoretical model and the prior literature.

Next, a process of iterative, collaborative program development should ensue, with members of the focal population helping to design and critique the intervention components. This iterative dialogue between planners and community members is vital to ensure that intervention materials are relevant, suitable, and engaging. In a review of HIV prevention interventions, Wilson and Miller (2003) found that interventionists relied on two strategies when developing culturally grounded programs. The first strategy was to attend to the intervention presentation by designing and presenting the intervention in such a manner that they appeal to the focal audience by including culturally specific facilitators, actors, images/icons, language/terminology, physical settings, and videos. The second strategy focused on culturally grounding the intervention content by addressing the experiences, values, and norms of the target group into the intervention content. Wilson and Miller's (2003) review suggested that the latter approach of integrating cultural concepts into programs was a more effective strategy than merely focusing on the presentation aspects of the program, highlighting the value of having community members offer their lived experience during the program design.

Cultural Tailoring of Pre-Packaged Interventions

Evidence-based interventions (EBIs) can provide public health departments and community agencies with helpful resources to use when attempting to promote the health and well-being of LGBTQ populations. The challenge in using EBIs is that they may not be transferrable to new populations or settings, as most have been designed, tailored, and evaluated for use with a specific population and community. When EBIs are being considered for use with another group and/or setting than originally intended, it is the responsibility of the program planner to examine the theoretical mechanisms of change proposed in the intervention and ascertain whether the strategies can be culturally tailored and/or adapted through the input of the community.

Cultural tailoring can occur at various levels (Resnicow, Baranowski, Ahluwalia, and Braithwaite 1999; Resnicow, Braithwaite, DiIorio, and Glanz 2002). The first is *surface structure*, which involves matching intervention materials and messages to observable social and behavioral characteristics of a focal population. This type of tailoring examines the extent to which the program fits with the culture, experience, and behavioral patterns of the audience. For example, using this approach you would create print and audiovisual materials using people, places, language, music, foods, brand names, locations, and clothing familiar to and preferred by the target audience. This approach also involves identifying the channels and settings that are most appropriate for delivery of messages and programs, and understanding characteristics of the behavior in question. In contrast, *deep structure* reflects how cultural, social, psychological, environmental, and historical factors influence health behaviors differently across diverse populations. It involves understanding how members of the focal population perceive the cause, course, and treatment of illnesses. It also involves understanding how the focal population perceives the determinants of specific health behaviors, and involves appreciation for how religion, family, society, economics, and the government, both in perception and in fact, influence the target behavior. For example, Matthews et al. (2013) developed an LGBTQ-specific smoking cessation program by culturally adapting the American Lung Association's Freedom from Smoking (ALA-FFS) curriculum. By taking the ALA-FFs program's cognitive and behavioral approaches and educational content, Matthews and colleagues tailored the program materials to reflect culture, norms, and beliefs about LGBTQ men and women and their smoking behaviors. These materials were informed by LGBTQ smoking-community members, a panel of LGBTQ health experts, a literature review, and from recommendations from existing tailored smoking cessation programs.

Once it is determined that there is a need and desire for your EBI, the cultural adaptation process can begin. Cultural adaptation parallels the intervention development process described above, including forming one or more advisory boards, identifying intervention components where cultural elements may be embedded, and assessing the acceptability and relevance of various intervention components by engaging participants in simulated intervention activities to gain their perspectives on the intervention. Once these data have been analyzed and discussed with appropriate advisory boards, the process of adaptation should begin and involve advice and input from the advisory boards. When conducting this adaptation process, it is important to maintain the core elements of the EBI in order to increase the likelihood that its effectiveness will be retained. This also may involve additional focus groups or pilot trials of various aspects of the intervention in order to gauge the appropriateness and acceptability of the new intervention components with your intended audience.

The last step is pilot testing the culturally adapted intervention (including all program materials) to ensure population acceptability and program implementation feasibility (Kettner, Moroney, and Martin 1999; Weiss 1998). Although community groups may not have the resources to do a full pilot, we recommend that every effort be made to test the intervention components (particularly if they are new and/or if the action board expressed concern or disagreement about specific content). Beyond the review of intervention materials, a pilot test can serve to solidify recruitment and retention plans, identify any foreseeable difficulties with the delivery of the intervention, and garner feedback on the program evaluation tools.

Summary and Next Steps. Programs and interventions might have components that are adapted from prior evidence-based interventions. The process of adaptation, however, will require program planners to understand the needs of their constituents and ensure that these programs are tailored to these communities. During the development of the program, attention should be given to who will deliver the intervention, as well as when and where these activities will take place. Often, program planners and community members will draft a program implementation plan to describe the resources necessary to carry out the intervention, the timing of intervention activities, and who will be responsible for their execution and oversight. Once finalized, the implementation plan might inform the recruitment of LGBTQ participants into the intervention (see chapter 11) and the design of the process and outcome evaluation plan (see chapter 14).

Conclusions

LGBTQ health promotion efforts need to be rooted in the realities of the populations and communities impacted, and they must be designed with consideration of the agencies where these interventions will be delivered. Interventions focused on LGBTQ populations should recognize how sociopolitical environments contribute to health disparities and seek to strengthen the communities' resources and assets while assisting to overcome risks and deficits (Merton 1972; Minkler and Wallerstein 2005). In this chapter, we highlighted how the use of participatory action research in the program planning process might be used to bring about social change by involving community stakeholders in the planning process as early as possible to draw on their expertise and to build interest and commitment. Participatory planning methods improve access to various sources of data, help contextualize the phenomena of interest, and subsequently identify and select the intervention strategies with greatest potential. Beyond intervention development on a specific health problem, the use of participatory methods is desirable when addressing LGBTQ issues as it may create and foster multisectoral relationships that move research into action in other domains. Participatory methods also promote social justice efforts by enhancing community participation in the social change process, and by enabling community members to gain power and control over their own lives.

We recognize that participatory methods can have challenges. For instance, a lack of awareness of proper research methods on the part of community members can introduce biases, random error, or breaches in ethics. When community members are both participants and researchers, there is the potential for selection biases, both self-selection and other participant selection. Additional challenges include problems with being an unbiased researcher regarding identification of problems, developing methodology, and implementing solutions. To address these challenges, it is important to train researchers on ethics, research design, procedures, troubleshooting, and avoiding biases. Similarly, it is important to develop and maintain channels for new community members to join the planning process. New voices can promote innovation, ensure that the program or intervention is not unintentionally excluding constituents, and minimize complacency. Encouraging multiple perspectives at all levels of analysis (personal, family, organization, community) can help reduce these potential biases and promote multi-disciplinary solutions to address LGBTQ health issues.

Overall, participatory action research's goal is to transform social reality through the empowerment of the participants. Each community will have its own characteristics, history, and power dynamics. The participatory planning process can help the team learn more about the communities being served while empowering members of the LGBTQ community to become active agents in research and intervention development. Community members can identify the problems affecting them, as well as offer insights into the most actionable and sustainable solutions. Furthermore, intervention activities might be perceived as more relevant and reflective of the actual experiences. We encourage program planners interested in designing LGBTQ interventions to leverage the rich historical tradition of LGBTQ advocacy and community participation and catalyze these efforts into strategies that create dialogue and advance public health practice.

References

Arnstein, S. R. 1969. A ladder of citizen participation. *Journal of the American Institute of Planners* 35(4): 216–24.

Bauermeister, J. A., Pingel, E. S., Sirdenis, T. J., Andrzejewski, J., Gillard, G., and Harper, G. W. on behalf of the Michigan Forward in Enhancing Research and Community Equity Coalition. 2017. Ensuring community participation during program planning: Lessons learned during the development of a HIV/STI program for young sexual and gender minorities. *American Journal of Community Psychology* 60(1–2): 215–18.

Bartholomew, L. K., Parcel, G. S., Kok, G., and Gottlieb, N. H. 2001. *Intervention Mapping: Designing Theory and Evidence-based Health Promotion Programs.* Mountain View, CA: Mayfield.

Bryant, L., Damarian, A. K., and Marshall, Z. 2014. Tobacco control recommendations identified by LGBT Atlantans in a community-based participatory research project. *Progress in Community Health Partnerships: Research, Education, and Action* 8: 269–79.

Carter, L., Hedges, L., and Congdon, S. 2012. Using diversity interventions to increase cervical screenings of lesbian and bisexual women. *Journal of Psychological Issues in Organizational Culture* 3(2): 59–71.

Dworkin, S. L., Pinto, R. M., Hunter, J., Rapkin, B., and Remien, R. H. 2008. Keeping the spirit of community partnerships alive in the scale up of HIV/AIDS prevention: Critical reflections on the roll out of DEBI (Diffusion of Effective Behavioral Interventions). *American Journal of Community Psychology* 42: 51–59.

Grov, C., Ventuneac A., Rendina, H. J., Jimenez, R. H., and Parsons, J. T. 2012 Perceived importance of five different health issues for gay and bisexual men: Implications for new directions in health education and prevention. *American Journal of Men's Health* 7(4): 274–84.

Harper, G. W., Bangi, A. K., Contreras, R., Pedraza, A., Tolliver, M., and Vess, L. 2004. Diverse phases of collaboration: Working together to improve community-based HIV interventions for youth. *American Journal of Community Psychology* 33(3/4): 193–204.

Harper, G. W., Contreras, R., Bangi, A., and Pedraza, A. 2003. Collaborative process evaluation. *Journal of Prevention & Intervention in the Community* 26: 53–69.

Institute of Medicine. 2011. *The Health of Lesbian, Gay, Bisexual, and Transgender People: Building a Foundation for Better Understanding*. Washington, DC: National Academies Press.

Israel, B. A., Schulz, A. J., Parker, E., and Becker, A. 1998. Review of community-based research: Assessing partnership approaches to improve public health. *Annual Review of Public Health* 19: 173–202.

Kettner, P. M., Moroney, R. M., and Martin, L. L. 1999. *Designing and Managing Pograms: An Effectiveness-Based Approach*. London: Sage Publications

MacQueen, K. M., McLellan, E., Metzger, D. S., Kegeles, S., Strauss, R. P., Scotti, R., . . . Trotter, R. T. 2001. What is community? An evidence-based definition for participatory public health. *American Journal of Public Health* 91: 1929–38.

Matthews, A., Li, C. C., Kuhns, L. M., Tasker, T. B., and Cesario, J. A. 2013. Results from a community-based smoking cessation treatment program for LGBT smokers. *Journal of Environmental and Public Health* 2013: 1–9,

McKenzie J. F, Neiger, B. L., and Thackeray R. 2013. *Planning, Implementing, and Evaluating Health Promotion Programs: A Primer*. San Francisco: Pearson

Merton, R. K. 1972. Insiders and outsiders: A chapter in the sociology of knowledge. *American Journal of Sociology* 78(1): 9–47.

Minkler, M., and Wallerstein, N. 2003. *Community-Based Participatory Research for Health: From Process to Outcomes*. San Francisco: Jossey-Bass.

Pachankis, J. E., Hatzenbuehler M. L., Rendina, H. J., Safren, S. A., and Parsons, J. T. 2015. LGB-affirmative cognitive-behavioral therapy for young adult gay and bisexual men: A randomized controlled trial of a transdiagnostic minority-stress approach. *Journal of Consulting and Clinical Psychology* 83(5): 875–89.

Resnicow, K., Baranowski, T., Ahluwalia, J. S., and Braithwaite, R. L. 1999. Cultural sensitivity in public health: Defined and demystified. *Ethnicity and Disease* 9(1): 10–21.

Ryan C., Russell, S. T., Huebner, D., Diaz, R., and Sanchez, J. 2010. Family acceptance in adolescence and the health of LGBT young adults. *Journal of Child and Adolescent Psychiatric Nursing* 23(4): 205–13.

Seelman, K. L., Adams, M. A., and Poteat, T. 2016. Interventions for healthy gaining among mature Black lesbians: Recommendations gathered through community-based research. *Journal of Women & Aging* 29(6): 530–42.

Senreich, E. 2010. Are specialized LGBT program components helpful for gay and bisexual men in substance abuse treatment? *Substance Use & Misuse* 46(7–8): 1077–96.

Suarez-Balcazar, Y., Harper, G. W., and Lewis, R. 2005. An interactive and contextual model of community-university collaborations for research and action. *Health Education & Behavior* 32(1): 84–101.

Wang, C., and Burris, M. 1997. Photovoice: Concept, methodology, and use for participatory needs assessment. *Health Education & Behavior* 24(3): 369–87.

Wang, C. C., Yi, W. K., Tao, Z. W., and Carovano, K. 1998. Photovoice as a participatory health promotion strategy. *Health Promotion International* 13: 75–86.

Zimmerman, M. A. 2000. Empowerment theory: Psychological, organizational, and community levels of analysis. In J. Rappaport and E. Seidman, eds., *Handbook of Community Psychology,* 43–63. New York: Kluwer Academic Publishers.

FOURTEEN

From Discovery to Application

Challenges in Effectiveness and Implementation Research for the Promotion of LGBTQ Health and Wellness

Robin Lin Miller and Angulique Y. Outlaw

> Learning is not attained by chance; it must be sought for with ardor and attended to with diligence.
>
> Abigail Adams

LGBTQ POPULATIONS too often experience poor health outcomes. Myriad factors drive elevated risk for cancer, mental illnesses, and other diseases among LGBTQ people, including low rates of health insurance coverage; high rates of stress due to systematic harassment, discrimination, and stigma; and the lack of culturally sensitive health care. As a consequence, LGBTQ people are more likely to smoke, drink alcohol, use illicit drugs, and engage in risky behaviors that can lead to sexually transmitted infections (Krehely 2009; Committee on Lesbian, Gay, Bisexual, and Transgender Health Issues and Research Gaps and Opportunities 2011). LGBTQ people who are members of racial or ethnic minority populations or who are of low income may be especially vulnerable to these negative health outcomes. The benefits of reducing health disparities among LGBTQ populations include promoting their wellness and longevity, curtailing disease transmission and progression, and reducing unnecessary health care costs (Krehely 2009; Office of Disease Prevention and Health Promotion 2016).

In this chapter, we address the key research issues in moving promising public health and wellness interventions out of the planning and development stages and into routine use for the benefit of LGBTQ people. We highlight the unique issues confronting public health research as it seeks to transfer its very best ideas from the laboratory to the realm of day-to-day practice. We contend that evidence-supported interventions (ESIs) must ultimately be judged by their performance on the ground in the hands of ordinary practitioners serving LGBTQ communities and by their ability to produce effects that are powerful enough, once institutionalized, to be of practical benefit to LGBTQ people.

Efficacy and Effectiveness Trials

Most health promotion research frameworks conceive of intervention research in stages. Prior chapters in this book detail the early research phases required to craft an intervention that promises to improve health outcomes. Determining whether a promising intervention actually contributes to population health defines the next research phase. Promising interventions typically undergo efficacy and effectiveness testing following the formative phases of their development. *Efficacy trials* seek to determine whether interventions produce expected results under ideal (controlled and adequately resourced) circumstances (Flay et al. 2005; Institute of Medicine 1994). *Effectiveness trials* examine the results that are likely to be observed under real-life conditions. In both cases, experimental approaches that permit confident causal attributions are considered the gold standard, with strong quasi-experimental designs comprising acceptable alternatives when true experiments prove too costly or infeasible.

Efficacy Trials

Efficacy trials (*explanatory trials*) provide evidence that an intervention produces a desired effect under carefully controlled conditions. Successfully designing and implementing these trials takes tremendous resources, diligence, and expertise to preserve the internal validity of the trial. The high demands of efficacy trials often necessitate that they occur in settings with well-developed capacity for executing complex research. Efficacy trials additionally require extensive training and staff supervision, diligent monitoring of intervention delivery for fidelity, and incentivized participation of trial participants. Although these strategies circumvent potential threats to internal validity, they have also resulted in criticism as they increase threats to both external and social validity due to limited generalizability outside of a trial setting.

Sampling and recruitment issues require extra attention in conducting efficacy trials. The populations that are recruited to participate in efficacy trials almost always differ from the people who stand to benefit the most from the intervention being tested. Bickman and Reich (2015) note, for example, that the people who are enrolled in efficacy trials for cancer treatment are typically healthier and younger than the normative cancer patient. We know of no research on the extent to which efficacy trial participants are representative of LGBTQ populations as a whole or include adequate sample sizes of those in the LGBTQ community with the greatest need. Research on the nature of funded studies targeting LGBTQ people strongly suggests the possibility that health-related efficacy trials infrequently target LGBTQ people and may not include those subpopulations that are most vulnerable to adverse health outcomes (Coulter et al. 2014). Although general population trials might include LGBTQ people, many of these efforts fail to assess participants' sexual and gender identity, precluding the possibility of decomposing intervention effects for LGBTQ participants.

Efficacy trials eliminate selection bias through randomization procedures. However, eliminating systematic selection bias requires samples that are sufficiently large to distribute potentially biasing characteristics evenly across research conditions. For trials that focus on LGBTQ people specifically, the ability to recruit an adequately large sample of LGBTQ people to eliminate selection threats may be difficult to achieve. Recruitment may be additionally hampered by reluctance to reveal LGBTQ identity to researchers. For efficacy trials, this presents a Catch-22. Recruiting sufficient numbers of LGBTQ people to run a trial may require operating that trial where recruitment is possible, limiting the generalizability of the results to the larger population of LGBTQ people who do not reside in areas dense with LGBTQ people who are out, motivated to participate in research, and able to meet the demanding expectations of trial participation. In combination, relatively small sample sizes for LGBTQ-specific trials, bias in the inclusion of diverse LGBTQ subpopulations, and lack of routine collection of information on LGBTQ participants in general population trials limit the extent to which the efficacy of many interventions for addressing LGBTQ health concerns can be determined.

Effectiveness Trials

Effectiveness trials (*pragmatic trials*) determine whether an intervention can reproduce the results observed in efficacy trials under circumstances that are believed to be representative of the real world (e.g., clinical practice) (Venere 2014; Bowen et al. 2009). By intent, effectiveness trials allow for some natural variation of the kind that is likely to occur under ordinary circumstances. For instance, researchers implementing effectiveness trials are often less concerned with exerting precise control over fidelity of implementation than those conducting an efficacy trial. Loosened controls in an effectiveness trial allow researchers to learn how difficult fidelity will be to achieve and how much variation in fidelity they can expect to observe once the ESI is carried out under real-world conditions. Regrettably, effectiveness trials bring with them similar demands as efficacy studies, plus additional resource demands, which make these trials exceedingly rare.

Implementation scholar Russell Glasgow and his colleagues note that effectiveness trials typically require enlisting as research partners multiple provider settings of the kind that are most likely to carry out an intervention (Glasgow, Lichtenstein, and Marcus 2003). By default, effectiveness trials require assessing the effects of interventions that have performed well in efficacy trials in settings characterized by varying degrees of capability to participate in research. Effectiveness trials may end up relying on a nonrepresentative subset of providers who possess unique capabilities and resources for the trial to proceed smoothly. The results of the trial may be biased as a consequence of relying on non-representative provider settings in order for the work to be accomplished. For LGBTQ effectiveness trials, this may mean that effectiveness trials favor assessing effects at premier institutions known for their research capability, ability to recruit desired subpopulations of LGBTQ participants, and competence in working with LGBTQ populations. Whether these settings are truly representative of the range of places where interventions might ultimately be implemented and whether these exist in sufficient number to replicate findings in multiple trial efforts is unknown.

Not every good idea for an intervention or every efficacious intervention will prove itself feasible and acceptable. Effectiveness research is especially useful for identifying whether an intervention is likely to prove feasible to implement in diverse settings and acceptable to providers and target populations prior to a scale-up effort. Obtaining findings to identify the probable generalizability of an intervention to diverse LGBTQ health providers and constituents represents a key challenge for effectiveness trials. Although the terms "feasibility" and "acceptability" are often used interchangeably, each has distinct meaning (Hindocha et al. 2013; Bowen et al. 2009). *Feasibility* refers to an intervention's practicality for being conducted in the field—whether the logistics of implementing it are workable. *Acceptability* refers to how well the intervention is received by the target population. Investigating both feasibility and acceptability matters, as effectiveness trials help to determine whether modifications to an intervention might need to be made and whether attempting to disseminate the intervention is worthwhile.

Inclusion of LGBTQ perspectives in the design and conduct of effectiveness trials may simultaneously lessen any distrust held by LGBTQ populations to research involvement and increase the possibility of creating an effectiveness trial that provides a sound indication of how likely it is that an intervention can reach LBGT communities (Ayala and Elder 2011). The same research methods used to aid in developing an intervention (e.g., observations, interviews, focus groups) may be useful for assessing whether prospective users and intended beneficiaries find it feasible and acceptable.

Summary. Promising interventions must make the transition from demonstrating their efficacy to demonstrating their effectiveness prior to dissemination and scale-up. Both types of trials are necessary to decide whether broad dissemination of an intervention is worthwhile. Critical impediments to efficacy and effectiveness trial designs for LGBTQ health often revolve around issues of sampling. Principal challenges include obtaining adequate numbers of LGBTQ people to decompose effects (within general population trials) and to reduce selection biases. Ensuring sufficient diversity among LGBTQ trial participants may also prove challenging, given the nature and demands of trial participation. For effectiveness trials, enlisting an adequately representative sample of provider settings adds additional challenges. In trials implemented with the general population, sexual and gender identity often go unmeasured. Assessing sexual and gender identity as a routine practice might permit researchers to examine results for LGBTQ participants alone and to draw implications for LGBTQ health from these trials. Incorporating assessments of feasibility and acceptability may be especially helpful for refining promising interventions prior to their dissemination and for anticipating the inevitable implementation challenges that occur in moving interventions to scale.

Moving to Application

Once the efficacy and effectiveness of interventions are established through experimental efficacy and effectiveness research trials, public health researchers face a new and often vexing challenge: getting someone to use their intervention on a routine basis to benefit vulnerable populations. Unfortunately, no matter how carefully developed and thoroughly tested a prototype intervention might be, the people who might use it, the populations with whom they might use it, and the settings in which they might use it are by definition unique from the people and contexts in which the original intervention was created and tested. Moreover, although researchers are well practiced at disseminating what they know to one another at conferences and through academic journals, they often lack multiple, active, and direct relationships with prospective users. The often bemoaned chasm between scientifically supported interventions and ongoing practices in community settings frames the need for a public health research and evaluation agenda that seeks to: (1) identify effective approaches to *disseminating* ESIs to potential users, (2) inform appropriate *adaptations* and reinventions, and (3) describe the range of social and contextual factors that facilitate the sustained *implementation* of ESIs at a scale and level of quality sufficient to reduce health disparities and promote population health. These can prove daunting tasks for research and evaluation in general and are especially challenging within the context of LGBTQ health.

Dissemination and implementation processes and their attendant research activities are interventions into the day-to-day practices of service delivery systems. These complex and lengthy processes involve multiple actors occupying distinct roles. Although multiple dissemination and implementation models exist, none is specific to disseminating and implementing ESIs within the context of service provision to LGBTQ populations. Leading texts on dissemination and implementation research might address multiple types of human diversity but fail to address issues specific to sexual orientation and gender identity. Although these existing research models may provide insight on what to study in order to to achieve health outcomes and improved services for LGBTQ people, how best to apply these models in the context of LGBTQ health remains largely unexplored.

Dissemination

What good is a proven intervention if no one who might use it has heard of it? Dissemination research focuses on identifying best practices for communicating ESIs in order to encourage their adoption (Rabin and Brownson 2012). Among all of the areas of research and evaluation, from discovery to implementation, dissemination practices have received the greatest research attention (Dearing 2008). Even so, dissemination research too often remains an afterthought in the development of public health interventions (Ammerman, Smith, and Calancie, 2014).

Dissemination refers to an intentioned information-sharing process and, in this case, refers to information sharing among sets of actors who are connected in professional or practice networks serving LGBTQ people, the prospective users of ESIs. To disseminate an ESI through the professional networks of prospective users, intervention researchers must investigate how these communication networks operate and whom they include. Research across diverse settings and problem areas suggests that a key to ESI dissemination is identification of those who function as the natural advice-givers and key opinion-leaders in a professional network. The ideal opinion-leaders are linked to many other individuals who occupy structurally similar roles (Neal et al. 2011). Intervention researchers are not necessarily positioned as advice-givers to those who serve LGBTQ populations, at least not directly, nor are they in a structurally similar position (i.e., they do not work as managers and staff of community-based service programs, clinics, etc.). As Neal and colleagues (2015) note, researchers and practitioners often operate in worlds apart, with limited opportunities for interpersonal interaction and communication. Researchers are seldom part of the communication networks of the vast majority of prospective intervention users. A critical area for dissemination research, then, is to describe the communication and influence networks through which knowledge about ESIs might be shared.

Within the context of LGBTQ public health, dissemination requires an empirical analysis using techniques such as social network analysis, survey research, and focus groups of the dissemination networks through which providers who ordinarily address LGBTQ health learn about new practices. Network-oriented research can document the extent to which there are serviceable communication bridges between the community of scientists conducting public health intervention research, the professional purveyors of information on effective practices, and the individuals who are positioned on the front-lines of service delivery making daily decisions about how best to meet consumers' needs. In some cases, such as in large multiservice health organizations specializing in LGBTQ concerns (e.g., Fenway Health in Boston, Howard Brown Health Center in Chicago), researchers are a part of the organization and serve as boundary spanners for sharing this kind of information. In many other organizations, no similar research function exists. Information for prospective users on ESIs flowing into these organizations comes primarily from peer opinion leaders in other organizations and professional purveyor organizations, those for-profit and nonprofit providers and government entities created for the specific purpose of disseminating information (see, for example, the National LGBT Health Education Center at http://www.lgbthealtheducation.org/). Information on ESIs may also be shared through think tanks, advocacy organizations, and coalitions that focus on addressing specific health conditions or the needs of LGBTQ populations.

Research can establish who in a given professional network is considered influential in promoting the voluntary adoption of new ideas and practices. Determining who leads opinions on best practices and influences what others believe about innovations must be determined in order to know whom to target with information about any specific intervention. When these opinion-leaders are convinced of the merits of an ESI and are willing to serve as champions of its use, its uptake is more likely. For instance, organizations such as Howard Brown and Fenway Health may serve as flagships for their peer organizations. Peer organizations take notice when organizations such as these endorse a novel practice. Other organizations will pay the endorsements of these flagship organizations no mind.

Dissemination research is always specific to the audience of prospective users for a particular ESI and to the influence networks in which they are embedded. Different networks of prospective users exist for ESIs to assist gay and bisexual men cope with living with HIV infection, transgender women in quitting smoking, and lesbian breast cancer patients in achieving stress reduction during treatment. The prospective users of these three very different interventions are likely to operate in distinct, although perhaps overlapping, communities of practice. Awareness and uptake of these different programs may not be influenced by the same thought leaders.

Although LGBTQ-focused settings are critical locations for accessing service without discrimination and stigma related to LGBTQ-status or identity, LGBTQ people seek and receive services in nonspecialized settings ranging from the county health department to the local community hospital to urgent care to multiservice community centers. Some LGBTQ people may receive all of their care and services through non-LGBTQ-specialist institutions; this may be particularly true for LGBTQ people who are persons of color, live in nonurban areas, are economically disadvantaged, or experience their local LGBTQ center as marginalizing or stigmatizing by virtue of their race, ethnicity, or social class. Some LGBTQ people simply may not be out enough to want to seek services at an LGBTQ organization. The question of how to disseminate effective interventions of particular relevance to LGBTQ health broadly is especially troublesome. Are LGBTQ-specialized providers and their non-LGBTQ-specialized counterparts connected to one another? To what degree? The optimal channels of influence to use to disseminate ESIs for LGBTQ health, especially in the context of non-LGBTQ public health settings, have seldom been explored.[1]

The channels of greatest influence on specialized-LGBTQ providers are likely to differ from those influencing decisionmaking in nonspecialized settings. LGBTQ-focused providers reflect the mission to serve their constituencies in ways that may attune them to information on effective public health interventions for conditions affecting LGBTQ populations. Within the context of nonspecialized care provision, providers may be simultaneously unaware of the unique needs of LGBTQ populations and perceive specialized interventions targeted solely at LGBTQ people as of little or no relevance (Sherman, Kauth, Shipherd, and Street 2015; Hughes, Harolds, and Boyer, 2011). Failure to perceive LGBTQ people as especially vulnerable to particular public health problems may preclude providers from recognizing the possible benefits of proven interventions to their consumers. An important role for dissemination research in LGBTQ health includes how best to gain the attention of providers in nonspecialized settings.

Dissemination research also identifies the ideal mechanisms for disseminating information about ESIs to prospective users and barriers to their adoption decisions.[2] Empirically informed dissemination interventions can be designed to promote understanding of a particular ESI or to assist prospective users with selecting the best ESI to adopt for their particular needs. Dissemination interventions typically rely on social marketing and mass-media strategies, creating guidebooks and manuals, and offering technical assistance and training programs of varying length and intensity. Interventions may also guide users through the process of making appropriate ESI selections from a menu of options. The body of evidence to guide selection of dissemination interventions for various user types and contexts lags behind their creation. Comparative effectiveness research on best practices for reaching LGBTQ-specialty and nonspecialty providers is an important area for future investigation.

One increasingly popular mechanism calls for co-design of new programs and practices in partnership with prospective users. Co-design has the advantage of integrating users' perspectives, experiences of providing services, and knowledge of the constraints of their settings into the design from the outset (Alcaraz et al. in press; see chapter 13). Co-design has the benefit of including LGBTQ people when LGBTQ people are prospective users of an ESI. Co-design creates parity between research and LGBTQ communities and may facilitate ownership of the resulting ESI. Co-design may enhance the relevance of an ESI to consumers' lives. Co-design is an ethical imperative in some contexts, such as within tribal communities, which are sovereign nations.

Empirical investigation is required to identify the ideal communication strategy for each homogenous segment of a dissemination effort's audience, as each prospective audience of users often requires a unique message targeting their particular values and concerns, and delivered via a tailored strategy with which they are comfortable and familiar (Storey, Saffitz and Rimon 2008). Some LGBTQ providers, for example, may be especially responsive to program features such as an emphasis on LGBTQ empowerment or an LGBTQ strengths-oriented perspective. These same values may not be prioritized by a provider who does not possess a unique focus on LGBTQ populations and for whom applicability across multiple other human diversities is a greater concern. Values prioritized in low-resourced organizations serving disadvantaged LGBTQ populations may differ markedly from those prioritized in well-resourced organizations. Although a knowledge base of efficient and effective approaches for disseminating ESIs to the diversity of LGBTQ providers is sorely needed, several excellent examples of dissemination programs for specific ESIs are available as models (see, for example, the multiple-year dissemination and intervention research effort conducted by Susan Kegeles and colleagues to disseminate the MPowerment Project).

Summary. For LGBTQ health, lack of dissemination research specific to LGBTQ service provision may impede the uptake of ESIs across diverse disease areas. Lack of knowledge of health disparities affecting LGBTQ populations may also impede dissemination to nonspecialized providers. Although specialist LGBTQ health and community service providers are common in many urban settings, LGBTQ populations also access services in nonspecialized environments. Dissemination of ESIs will be enhanced through research to document the professional networks of LGBTQ service provision, user segmentation studies of providers in these networks, studies of factors that influence decisions to adopt or reject ESIs, and inclusion of prospective adopters in the co-design of promising interventions. Social network investigations, comparative effectiveness studies of dissemination strategies, and mixed methods approaches to guide message framing and content can improve existing knowledge on how to disseminate ESIs to improve LGBTQ health.

Adaptation

Although a small number of ESIs have been developed specifically for LGBTQ people, most public health ESIs were not. Only 698 studies (0.1%) funded by the National Institutes of Health (NIH) over a 23-year period addressed LGBTQ health concerns (Coulter et al. 2014). Of these, the vast majority (75%) focused on HIV; of 202 NIH-funded LGBTQ intervention studies, 181 (89.6%) addressed HIV-related issues. No LGBTQ intervention studies were funded in important health areas including maternal and infant health, exercise and physical activity, nutrition, diabetes, oral health, and cardiovascular disease. As a consequence of the attention given to HIV, nearly all of the intervention studies on LGBTQ health targeted gay and bisexual men (n=182). Only 15 intervention studies focused on transgender people and 12 on lesbian and bisexual women (Coulter et al. 2014). These data suggest that many subgroups of LGBTQ people are normatively excluded from the most rigorous program of health-focused intervention research in the United States. Moreover, even when LGBTQ people are the principal focus, not every intervention study will lead to a program or practice earning the status of an ESI.

Community-developed interventions exist in multiple disease and wellness areas targeting LGBTQ populations (Nieves-Lugo et al. 2016). These interventions may possess certain advantages because of their community and practice-based origins, including being designed with an eye toward implementation feasibility and community acceptability. But community-developed programs have often not been sufficiently evaluated (Miller and Shinn 2005; Miller 2003). Without rigorous evaluations, the evidence on the typical community-developed program may not meet the standards scientists, clearinghouses, and government entities apply when labeling an intervention evidence-supported.

As a consequence of these two trends—the normative exclusion of LGBTQ people from diverse public health intervention research and limited evaluation of community-developed interventions—in nearly every area of public health and wellness, adopting an ESI to meet the health needs of an LGBTQ population will require that the ESI be adapted. Adaptation refers to the process of modifying an ESI to fit local realities and consumers while preserving its core elements and guiding principles. Adaptations may occur in response to features of the user's setting and characteristics of its implementing staff, such as the size of available space, degree of autonomy granted to front-line workers, or the skill level and experience of the staff in delivering ESIs or working with the target population; features of the ESI, such as its level of complexity, its flexibility, and its specificity; and features of the intended target population, such as their age, sex, level of educational attainment, mobility, and severity of risk (Allen, Linnan, and Emmons 2012; Castor, Barrera, and Martinez 2004). Adaptations must often respond to all of these areas of concern in order to achieve adequate tailoring and produce a modified ESI that is conceptually equivalent, delivers the content suitably for its new audience, and provides content in a form that matches consumers' and staff's strengths, challenges, and needs.

For LGBTQ populations, ESIs may need to be adapted to respond to staff's attitudes, beliefs, skills, and experience in addressing LGBTQ concerns. For instance, instructions to facilitators may need to offer staff more specific and detailed guidance on culturally competent problem-solving in discussions, role plays, and exercises. Role plays may not reflect common experiences (Miller, Klotz, and Eckholdt 1998; Miller 2003). In some settings that may seem well positioned to offer an ESI targeting LGBTQ populations, staff may not all share affirming attitudes or be competent in and sufficiently familiar with LGBTQ consumers (Wilson et al. 2013). Target population adaptations for LGBTQ audiences might need to address such wide-ranging issues as cultural and religious beliefs, norms, and preferences; developmental appropriateness; regional or geographic matters; socio-economic considerations; literacy, numeracy, and health literacy; outness and willingness to identify as LGBTQ; the nature and severity of social and behavioral determinants of risk; and sources of resilience. As Garnets and Kimmel note (2003, 349), shared sexual and gender identity alone offers little guarantee that people will experience the world in common, suggesting the importance of adapting ESIs with refined sensitivity to LGBTQ relevance *and* LGBTQ diversity. What might LGBTQ-specific adaptations require? At a minimum, adaptations to language and imagery. ESIs may employ gender-binary and heteronormative language in handouts, exercises, and scripts. Adaptations might include replacing photographs of heterosexual couples with same-sex couples or replacing video or other stimulus materials. New intervention components may be needed to address the specific contribution of factors such as internalized homophobia, minority stress, and discriminatory experiences resulting from LGBTQ status.

A small number of formal models exist to guide adaptation research and may be readily tailored for use with LGBTQ populations (e.g., CDC's ADAPT model [McKleroy et al. 2006] and Wingood and DiClemente's ADAPT-ITT model [Wingood and DiClemente 2008]). Adaptation models emphasize empirically guided adaptations and thorough pilot-testing. Wingood and DiClemente, for example, advocate intensive data collection in the form of focus groups, qualitative interviews, and needs assessment activities with target population members and staff as the initial step to identify appropriate adaptations. Adaptation research rooted in transformative research paradigms may be particularly useful for eliciting diverse LGBTQ perspectives (Mertens 2009). Transformative paradigms emphasize placing the worldview of marginalized and underrepresented people at the fore in order to legitimate the experiences and promote socially just outcomes for people who lack social power. Transformative paradigms are consistent with the emancipatory and human rights orientation of many LGBTQ-focused community providers and are therefore well suited to adaptation research occurring in this context.

Summary. Finding the right balance between tailoring an ESI to a new target population and the setting in which they will be served and preserving the key ingredients that make the ESI effective can at times feel like walking a tightrope. Randomization and a focus on average effects purposefully obscure the significance of individual differences in the experimental research efforts that typically lead to the designation as an ESI. Studies often de-emphasize generalizability, leaving the applicability and relevance of ESIs to diverse populations and practice-based settings in doubt (Beecher and Trickett 2016; Green and Nasser 2012; Ammerman, Smith, and Calancie, 2014). The research required to tackle an adaptation successfully includes documenting the basic principles and theories underlying the ESI and laying out its core elements or key ingredients. With a thorough understanding of what makes a particular ESI effective, research can then be used to understand the constraints and resources in the new implementation context and to identify the relevant needs, perspectives, and experiences of the new target population. The potential for conflict between the culture, values, and assumptions embedded in an ESI and those groups to which ESIs might be adapted is heightened by inattention to settings, circumstances, and populations in efficacy and effectiveness research. Thorough adaptation research that elicits the opinions and views of LGBTQ populations is needed to ensure that ESIs are relevant to diverse LGBTQ communities and feasible to carry out in the settings in which LGBTQ people access services.

Implementation

In order to confer their public health benefits, ESIs must be carried out in a high-quality and sustained manner, yet many factors can undermine an ESI's quality and sustainment. Implementation research investigates the factors that support and undermine sustained use of ESIs in daily practice and the fidelity of their implementation over time.

Consumer Factors

Although it is an important consideration, there is a dearth of research on the consumer factors that may undermine or facilitate successful implementation of an ESI. As we previously noted, the consumers served by any one agency will differ in important ways from the people who participated in the original research activity leading to an ESI designation. Consumers may be more transient and have more complicated or multiple needs than the people who participated in the original trial. They may use services only intermittently and unpredictably. Consumers may not be especially responsive to an ESI because they perceive it as irrelevant or not the optimal approach to addressing their needs. These factors may create low levels of engagement in an ESI or make ongoing and stable recruitment and retention into ESIs difficult (Kegeles et al. 2015; Miller 2001). For LGBTQ populations, distrust or discomfort with the staff at the institution offering the ESI and prior experiences of discrimination, service refusal, bias, cultural incompetence, or humiliation may further undermine successful implementation.

User Factors

Individual beliefs and practice norms of workers influence implementation outcomes, including fidelity. When workers do not believe an ESI will benefit their consumers or perceive it as incompatible with their core values or approach to their work, they are less likely to carry it out. Providers may alter or eliminate elements of an ESI to fit their approach to practice (Owczarzak, Broaddus, and Pinkerton 2016).

LGBTQ-specific providers may possess longstanding ambivalence and distrust of intervention research, as they may feel that research has not always furthered the community's rights and dignity. ESIs may rest on a base of evidence that is perceived as pathologizing of LGBTQ people, inconsistent with an LGBTQ rights agenda, or insufficiently inclusive of the LGBTQ community in the process of knowledge production (Andrasick et al. 2014; Matthews et al. 2016). These distrustful and skeptical attitudes may be accentuated within the context of LGBTQ communities of color, who may feel alienated from and exploited by research and therefore inclined to reject its products. Among non-LGBTQ-specific providers, negative attitudes toward LGBTQ populations or unfamiliarity with them may undermine quality of implementation of regular services (Lamda Legal 2010) and create an environment with weak capability to implement ESIs with LGBTQ people successfully.

Setting Factors

Organizational characteristics and the larger geographic and political climate in which organizations exist may also undermine fidelity and sustained implementation (Kegeles et al. 2015; Miller et al. 2012; Owczarzak 2012; Veniegas, Kao, and Rosales 2009). LGBTQ-specific organizations often form because mainstream providers are perceived as indifferent to LGBTQ needs. Workers in these settings may be especially attuned to the relevance of particular ESIs, given their presumed community expertise. ESIs operating in place of or alongside staff-developed efforts may challenge staff's sense of population expertise, control, and autonomy, especially when the use of an ESI is imposed and leadership around its use is not strong and enduring.

Many LGBTQ-specific organizations are small and under-resourced (Miller 2017; Rotheram-Borus, Swendeman and Chorpita 2012). Small and under-resourced organizations are prone to turnover and instability, circumstances that undermine their ability to implement ESIs. For instance, turnover prompts the constant need for retraining. The costs of retraining staff in a complex ESI may rapidly outweigh the benefits in such a setting. Resource challenges may increase an organization's need for technical assistance on an ESI, while limiting their ability to take full advantage of implementation assistance. Ultimately, organizations may drop parts of ESIs, simplify them, or abandon them all together, opting for less costly and complex alternatives.

For LGBTQ-specific providers, geography matters. Outside of major urban settings, it may be especially difficult to access enough LGBTQ people to offer any particular ESI with frequency. There may be too few people who are willing and able to take advantage of an ESI more than occasionally, placing organizations at risk of failing to meet accountability expectations (Miller et al. 2011). Local competition among providers attempting to serve the same population, sometimes via the same ESI, can also undermine implementation. Given how few LGBTQ providers exist and how few ESIs there are specific to the population, it may not be unusual to find two versions of the same ESI being implemented miles apart, creating pressure on each organization to appear unique in filling a niche. Rural, conservative, and oppressive sociopolitical contexts might force LGBTQ organizations to keep their efforts at low profile, undermining their ability to reach their intended targets (Miller 2001). Implementation challenges arising from operating in this context might result in significant modifications to an ESI in order to complete basic processes such as consumer recruitment.

Ongoing evaluation plays a critical role in implementation. Implementation science and program evaluation overlap, although each rests on its own base of literature on theory, methods, and practice. Implementation science contributes to the development of general knowledge on organizational and contextual conditions supporting the successful use of ESIs in order to guide the design of intervention strategies to enhance implementation outcomes. By contrast, evaluation contributes to evidence-supported determinations of merit, worth, and significance in order to improve programs and inform decisions about them (Schwandt 2015). In the context of implementation, evaluation helps implementing staff members learn in real time.

Implementation evaluation focuses closely on what actually happens and captures the unforeseen conditions that affect how the plans for an ESI are carried out in reality (Patton 2008).[3] There are many types of implementation evaluation, including process evaluation, monitoring, and treatment specification. Regardless of the type, implementation evaluation provides feedback to staff to make midcourse corrections by identifying implementation problems and their sources and by providing an early assessment of the likelihood that desirable consequences will be achieved and undesirable consequences avoided. In this way, implementation evaluation ultimately prepares staff to demonstrate their efforts are worthwhile relative to criteria important to staff, consumers, and other stakeholders, and relative to the outcomes against which the original ESI's merit was established. Outcome evaluations use multiple criteria of merit reflecting multiple perspectives against which to arrive at evaluative judgements on merit and worth. Whereas implementation science focuses heavily on user experiences implementing ESIs, evaluation focuses heavily on consumer perceptions, experiences, and outcomes. Evaluation complements implementation research in part by highlighting consumer perspectives, as well as those of the intended consumers whom an ESI fails to reach. In the case of ESI implementation in the LGBTQ health context, evaluators might favor applying evaluation models that support social justice, inclusion, and empowerment.[4] Unfortunately, staff members often lack the time, investment, and expertise to produce and use evaluative evidence (Carman and Fredericks 2008). Resources to hire qualified external evaluators are often unavailable.[5]

Summary. Enthusiasm for the concept of scaling up effective approaches frequently overshadows critical reflection on when scale-up is warranted and feasible (Swerissen and Crisp 2004). Substantial evidence suggests calls to scale up ESIs may pay too little attention to the barriers and costs of bringing interventions to scale (Sarrafzadegan et al. 2014). Implementation research can aid in making decisions about when scale-up attempts are warranted and which are likely to succeed. ESIs that are shown to benefit populations in research demonstrations may not yield similar benefits in real-world conditions because of features of the intervention, of the populations an organization serves, of the implementing organization and its staff, or of the surrounding context. Implementation research can identify the factors that are most likely to influence an implementation effort for a particular ESI and that are pertinent to its being conducted successfully for LGBTQ people. Coupled with ongoing evaluation to support staff's learning and improvement, implementation research can enhance the probability of successful implementation outcomes. Qualitative and mixed-method approaches are ideally suited to implementation research and evaluation with LGBTQ populations. Involving LGBTQ communities in implementation research and evaluation in a meaningful fashion and in ways that are safe, respectful, and responsive to their needs, concerns, and experiences can be challenging. Yet community members' involvement helps to ensure that implementation science and evaluation adequately and credibly represent their values, perspectives, and needs.

Scaling to International Context

We have addressed key issues in moving an intervention through the phases of efficacy and effectiveness testing, dissemination, adoption, adaptation, and implementation within the context of the United States. What about scaling up programs internationally? Several factors merit particular attention when bringing ESIs for LGBTQ health to scale in other country contexts.

Expanding access to ESIs may be easy in countries that protect against discrimination based on LGBTQ status and that are culturally and economically similar to the countries in which an ESI was originally conceived. Unfortunately, these kinds of settings may not be the ones with the greatest need for ESIs targeting LGBTQ health or where the greatest health disparities exist. LGBTQ stigma manifests in entirely different ways in different national contexts. Whereas bias and discrimination affects LGBTQ people globally, seventy countries criminalize same-sex sexual contact; in six, people may be put to death for engaging in homosexual activity. Others imprison LGBTQ people. Even if anti-homosexuality laws are not in place or enforced, anti-gay rhetoric, prejudice, and discrimination against LGBTQ people may be widespread. Extreme stigma of this kind severely limits access to health care and other services, drives disparities for LGBTQ people, and may force LGBTQ populations to interact with providers only when it is necessary or without any disclosure and acknowledgment of LGBTQ status.

In political and social climates in which LGBTQ discrimination is prevalent and especially when discrimination and prejudice are legally sanctioned, the people who are positioned to provide services may be prone to accept the dominant societal stance. Staff—the prospective users of ESIs—managers, supervisors, and other decisionmakers may view LGBTQ people with disdain and perceive it is socially and morally just to deny them medical and other services. For instance, in a recently published study of roughly 4,000 Nigerian young adults, more than a third of respondents indicated gay men ought to be denied medical care (Sekoni et al. 2016). ESIs for LGBTQ people may encounter cultural hostility that manifests in resistance to adoption and implementation. ESIs may also risk fanning a backlash at the imposition of foreign systems of beliefs and values on the local culture.

LGBTQ-specific ESIs may take for granted that consumers exist in environments that are at least tolerant of LGBTQ status and in which they are freed from legal sanction and institutionalized discrimination. As this may not be the case in many country contexts, anti-bias and discrimination interventions may need to accompany dissemination and adaptation efforts in order to secure buy-in, counter biases and stigmatizing beliefs, and develop staff competence and skill in serving LGBTQ people. Attention may also need to be given to any risks that staff may incur for implementing an LGBTQ-focused ESI and to protecting consumers' privacy and safety. ESIs may need to add components to address violence and structural factors that increase risk for LGBTQ community members, as these may undermine sustained implementation (Maiorana et al. 2016). Recruitment of LGBTQ people into ESIs may be especially fraught in settings in which LGBTQ people feel compelled to conceal same-sex attractions in order to avoid social and legal sanctions. Specialized recruitment and intervention delivery mechanisms appropriate to the protection of consumers and to the norms in the setting regarding socializing among LGBTQ people may need to be devised.

Whether a country is high in its stigma of LGBTQ people or is more tolerant, cultural differences and the culturally embedded assumptions in ESIs will require explicit examination in order for ESIs to be adapted to reflect life on the ground for LGBTQ people in all its complexity (see, for example, Maiorana et al. 2016). At a minimum, ESIs must be per-ceived as culturally acceptable to consumers and implementing users (Pallas et al. 2013). In addition to ensuring a culturally compatible ESI that reflects local LGBTQ experiences, local ownership and support of the ESI are likely to influence its long-term implementation (Hodge and Turner 2016).

Service delivery cultures and resources merit close investigation too. In many low- and middle-income country environments, the baseline level of system preparedness to provide services and the resources to support service provision are well below those of the high-income coun-tries in which ESIs are typically developed and tested initially. Certain ESIs may not be suitable to implementation in contexts characterized by weak infrastructure, financial strain, poorly trained staff, and inad-equate physical space. Careful assessment of resource compatibility to establish the feasibility of implementing particular ESIs may be needed.

Conclusions

LGBTQ people are too seldom identified in efficacy and effectiveness trials or the subject of large trials with adequate replication studies. There is a dearth of research on how providers who might serve LGBTQ people are structured into communities of practice and on the nature of their communication networks.[6] We know very little about who influ-ences beliefs and perceptions regarding the practices and programs that are viewed by service providers as feasible, effective, and culturally appro-priate to diverse LGBTQ populations. Adaptations of ESIs to LGBTQ people are seldom studied, as are implementation efforts of ESIs target-ing LGBTQ people. As such, we know too little about how to maximize the benefits of ESIs to support LGBTQ health.

Dissemination and implementation research efforts are urgently needed to identify appropriate targets of dissemination for LGBTQ ESIs, map the connections among these institutions, and identify natural pat-terns of dissemination of ideas among them. Research might also iden-tify what kinds of providers are commonly and uncommonly repre-sented in these networks in terms of the subpopulations they serve. The latter is essential for reducing disparities that occur within LGBTQ communities, as it may suggest distinct channels of influence to bring ESIs to people of distinct incomes, racial and ethnic backgrounds, and geographic locations. A robust program of research on the adaptations necessary to create ESIs that are effective, feasible, scalable, and relevant is also needed. Coupled with an effort to examine implementation domestically and abroad, we can maximize the potential of ESIs to improve LGBTQ health globally.

Notes

1. There are published efforts to create LGBT health centers within settings such as hospitals that offer useful guidance, but these studies do not address adoption, uptake, and implementation of ESIs per se.

2. Multiple formal dissemination and implementation models among which one might select are articulated in the literature, including models specific to translating programs and practices to address mental health, addiction, and HIV/AIDS. The research base regarding the success of these models for translating evidence-supported interventions to LGBT health settings remains largely unexplored.

3. Patton (2008, 323–27) lists five implementation evaluation options: (1) effort, (2) monitoring, (3) process, (4) component, and (5) treatment specification.

4. In addition to Mertens's Transformative Evaluation approach, other approaches include Jennifer Greene's values-engaged approach, David Fetterman's Empowerment Evaluation, House and Howe's Democratic Deliberative Evaluation, and an emerging number of culturally responsive evaluation techniques.

5. The American Evaluation Association has a topical interest group on GBLT issues in evaluation. The group has posted 31 publicly available posts on evaluating with LGBT populations at http://aea365.org/blog/category/lesbian-gay-bisexual-transgender-issues/.

6. A small number of studies examine interorganizational collaboration within the context of HIV care; for example, Jain, Maulsby, Kinsky, Khosla, Charles, Riordan, and Holtgrave (2016) report on the linkage-to-care networks in four US cities.

References

Alcaraz, K. I., Sly, J. Ashing, K. Fleisher L., Gil-Rivas, V. Ford, S. . . . and Gwede, C. K.. 2017. The ConNECT Framework: A model for advancing behavioral medicine science and practice to foster health equity. *Journal of Behavioral Medicine* 40(1): 23–38

Allen, J. D., Linnan, L. A., and Emmons, K. M. 2012. Fidelity and its relationship to implementation effectiveness, adaptation, and dissemination. In R. C. Brownson, G. A. Colditz, E. K. Proctor, ed., *Dissemination and Implementation Research in Health: Translating Science to Practice*, 281–304. New York: Oxford University Press.

Ammerman, A., Smith, T. W., and Calancie, L. 2014. Practice-based evidence in public health: Improving reach, relevance, and results. *Annual Review of Public Health* 35: 47–63.

Andrasick, M. P., Chandler, C. P., Wakefield, S., Kripke, K., and Eckstein, D. 2014. Bridging the divide: HIV prevention research and Black men who have sex with men. *American Journal of Public Health* 104(4): 708–14.

Ayala, G. X., and Elder, J. P. 2011. Qualitative methods to ensure acceptability of behavioral and social interventions to the target population. *Journal of Public Health Dentistry* 71(1): S69–S79.

Beecher, S., and Trickett, E. J. 2016. Community psychology misdirected? The case of evidence-based interventions. In M. A. Bond, I. Serrano-Garcia, and C. B. Keys, eds., *APA Handbook of Community Psychology, 1: Theoretical Foundations, Core Concepts, and Emerging Challenges,* 455–68. Washington, DC: American Psychological Association.

Bickman, L., and Reich, S. M. 2015. Randomized controlled trials: A gold standard or gold plated? In S. I. Donaldson, C. A. Christie, and M. M. Mark, eds., *Credible and Actionable Evidence: The Foundation for Rigorous and Influential Evaluations,* 83–113. Newbury Park: Sage.

Bowen, D. J., Kreuter, M., Spring, B., Cofta-Woerpel, L., Linnan, L., Weiner, D., . . . and Fernandez, M. 2009. How we design feasibility studies. *American Journal of Preventive Medicine* 36(5): 452–57.

Carman, J. G., and Fredericks, K. A. 2008. Nonprofits and evaluation: Empirical evidence from the field. *New Directions for Evaluation* 119: 51–71.

Castor, F. G., Barrera M., Jr., and Martinez, C. R., Jr., 2004. The cultural adaptation of prevention interventions: Resolving tensions between fidelity and fit. *Prevention Science* 5(1): 41–45.

Committee on Lesbian, Gay, Bisexual, and Transgender Health Issues and Research Gaps and Opportunities; Board on the Health of Select Populations; Institute of Medicine. 2011. Introduction. In *The Health of Lesbian, Gay, Bisexual, and Transgender People: Building a Foundation for Better Understanding,* 89–140. Washington, DC: National Academies Press.

Coulter, R. W., Kenst, K. S., Bowen, D. J., and Scout. 2014. Research funded by the National Institutes of Health on the health of lesbian, gay, bisexual, and transgender populations. *American Journal of Public Health* 104(2): e105–e112.

Dearing, J. W. 2008. Evolution of diffusion and simmeniation theory. *Journal of Public Health Management and Practice* 14(2): 99–108.

Flay, B. R., Biglan, A., Boruch, R. F., Castro, F. G., Gottfredson, D. C., and Kellam, S. 2005. Standards of evidence: Criteria for efficacy, effectiveness, and dissemination. *Prevention Science* 6(3): 451–74.

Garnets, L. D., and Kimmel, D. C. 2003. *Psychological Persepctives on Lesbian, Gay, and Bisexual Experiences,* 2nd ed. New York: Columbia University Press.

Glasgow, R. E., Lichtenstein, E., and Marcus, A. C. 2003. Why don't we see more translation of health promotion research to practice? Rethinking the efficacy-to-effectiveness transition. *American Journal of Public Health* 93(8): 1261–67.

Green, L. W., and Nasser, M. 2012. Furthering dissemination and implementation research: The need for more attention to external validity. In R. C. Brownson, G. A. Colditz, & E. K. Proctor, *Dissemination and Implementation Resarch in Health: Translating Science to Practice,* 305–26. New York: Oxford University Press.

Hindocha, S., Charlton, T., Rayment, M., and Theobald, N. 2013. Feasibility and acceptability of routine human immunodeficiency virus testing in general practice: Your views. *Primary Health Care Research and Development* 14(2): 212–16.

Hodge, L. M., and Turner, K. M. 2016. Sustained implementation of evidence-based programs in disadvantaged communities: A conceptual framework of supporting factors. *American Journal of Community Psychology* 58(1–2): 192–210.

Hughes, A. K., Harold, R. D., and Boyer, J. M. 2011. Awareness of LGBT issues among aging services network providers. *Journal of Gerentological Social Work* 54(7): 659–77.

Institute of Medicine. 1994. *Reducing Risks for Mental Disorders: Frontiers for Preventive Intervention Research*. Washingon DC: National Academies Press.

Jain, K. M., Maulsby, C., Kinsky, S., Khosla, N., Charles, V., Riordan, M., and Holtgrave, D. R. 2016. Exploring changes in interagency collaboration following AIDS United's Positive Charge: A five-site HIV linkage and retention in care program. *Health Education and Behavior* 46(3): 674–82.

Kegeles, S. M., Rebchook, G., Tebbetts, S., and Arnold, E. 2015. Facilitators and barriers to effective scale-up of an evidence-based multi-level HIV prevention intervention. *Implementation Science* 10: article 50

Krehely, J. December 21, 2009. *How to Close the LGBT Health Disparities Gap*. Retrieved from Center for American Progress: https://www.americanprogress.org /issues/lgbt/reports/2009/12/21/7048/how-to-close-the-lgbt-health-disparities-gap/

Lambda Legal. 2010. *When Health Care Isn't Caring: Lambda Legal's Survey of Discrimination against LGBT People and People with HIV*. New York: Lambda Legal.

Maiorana, A., Kegeles, S., Salazar, X., Konda, K., Silva-Santisteban, A., and Caceres, C. 2016. "Proyecto Orgullo": An HIV prevention, empowerment and community mobilisation intervention for gay men and transgender women in Callao/ Lima, Peru. *Global Public Health* 11(7–8): 1076–92.

Matthews, D. D., Smith, J. C., Brown, A. L., and Malenbranche, D. J. 2016. Reconciling epidemiology and social justice in the public health discourse around the sexual networks of Black men who have sex with men. *American Journal of Public Health* 106(5): 808–14.

McKleroy, V. S., Galbraith, J. S., Cummings, B., Jones, P., Harshbarger, C., Collins, C., . . . Carey, J. W. 2006. Adapting evidence-based behavioral interventions for new settings and target populations. *AIDS Education and Prevention* 18(4 Supp. A): S59–S73.

Mertens, D. M. 2009. *Transformative Research and Evaluation*. New York: Guilford Press.

Miller, R. L. 2001. Innovation in HIV prevention: Organizational and intervention characteristics affecting program adoption. *American Journal of Community Psychology* 29(4): 621–47.

Miller, R. L. 2003. Adapting an evidence-based intervention: Tales of the Hustler Project. *AIDS Education and Prevention* 15(1 Supp. A): S127–S138.

Miller, R. L. 2017. Evaluating HIV-related practices and evidence-supported programs in AIDS community-based organizations. In R. Hopson, F. Cram, and R. Millett, *Evaluation in Complex Ecologies*. Palo Alto: Stanford University Press.

Miller, R. L., and Shinn, M. 2005. Learning from communities: Overcoming difficulties in dissemination of prevention promotion efforts. *American Journal of Community Psychology* 35(3–4): 169–83.

Miller, R. L., Forney, J. C., Hubbard, P., and Camacho, L. M. 2012. Reinventing Mpowerment for Black men: Long-term community implementation of an evidence-based program. *American Journal of Community Psychology* 49(1–2): 199–214.

Miller, R. L., Klotz, D., and Eckholdt, H. M. 1998. HIV prevention with male prostitutes and patrons of hustler bars: Replication of an HIV prevention intervention. *American Journal of Community Psychology* 26(1): 97–131.

Miller, R. L., Levine, R. L., Khamarko, K., and Valenti, M. T. 2011. A dynamic model of client recruitment and retention in community-based HIV prevention. *Health Promotion Practice* 12(1): 135–46.

Neal, J. W., Neal, Z. P., Atkins, M. S., Henry, D. B., and Frazier, S. L. 2011. Channels of change: Contrasting network mechanisms in the use of interventions. *American Journal of Community Psychology* 47(3–4): 277–86.

Neal, Z. P., Neal, J. W., Lawlor, J. A., and Mills, K. J. 2015. Small worlds or worlds apart? Using network theory to understand the research-practice gap. *Psychosocial Intervention* 24(3): 177–84.

Nieves-Lugo, K., Rohrbeck, C. A., Nakamura, N., and Zea, M. C. 2016. Interventions with lesbian, gay, bisexual, transgender, and questioning communities. In M. A. Bond, I. Serrano-Garcia, and C. B. Keys, *APA Handbook of Community Psychology*, 2: *Methods for Community Research and Action for Diverse Groups and Issues*, 555–69. Washington, DC: American Psychological Association.

Office of Disease Prevention and Health Promotion (US Department of Health and Human Services). October 10, 2016. *Lesbian, Gay, Bisexual, and Transgender Health*. Retrieved from Healthy People 2020: https://www.healthypeople.gov/2020/topics-objectives/topic/lesbian-gay-bisexual-and-transgender-health

Owczarzak, J. 2012. Evidence-based HIV prevention in community settings: Provider perspectives on evidence and effectiveness. *Critical Public Health* 22(1): 73–84.

Owczarzak, J., Broaddus, M., and Pinkerton, S. 2016. A qualitative analysis of the concepts of fidelity and adaptation in the implementation of an evidence-based HIV prevention intervention. *Health Education Research* 31(2): 283–94.

Pallas, S. W., Minhas, D., Perez-Escamilla, R., Taylor, L., Curry, L., and Bradley, E. H. 2013. Community health workers in low- and middle-income countries: What do we know about scaling up and sustainability? *American Journal of Public Health* 103(7): e74–e82.

Patton, M. Q. 2008. *Utilization-Focused Evaluation*, 4th ed. Newbury Park: Sage.

Rabin, B. A., and Brownson, R. C. 2012. Developing the terminology for dissemination and implementation research. In R. C. Brownson, G. A. Colditz, and E. K. Proctor, *Dissemination and Implementation Research in Health: Translating Science to Practice*, 23–51. New York: Oxford University Press.

Reed, S. J., and Miller, R. L. 2011. Identity and agency: The meaning and value of pregnancy for young Black lesbians. *Psychology of Women Quarterly* 34(4): 571–81.

Reed, S. J., Miller, R. L., Valenti, M. T., and Timm, T. M. 2011. Baby's daddies, dick dykes, and good gay females: Black lesbian community norms and the acceptability of pregnancy. *Culture, Health, and Sexuality* 13(7): 751–65.

Rotheram-Borus, M. J., Swendeman, D., and Chorpita, B. F. 2012. Disruptive innovations for designing and diffusing evidence-based interventions. *American Psychologist* 67(6): 463–76.

Schwandt, T. A. (2015). *Evaluation Foundations Revisited: Cultivating a Life of the Mind for Practice*. Palo Alto: Stanford University Press.

Sekoni, A. O., Jolly, K., Gale, N. K., Ifaniyi, O. A., Somefun, E. O., Agaba, E. I., and Fakayode, V. A. 2016. Provision of services to men who have sex with men in

Nigeria: Students' attitudes following the passage of the same-sex marriage prohibition law. *LGBT Health* 3(4): 300–307.

Sherman, M. D., Kauth, M. R., Shipherd, J. C., and Street, R. L., Jr. 2014. Provider beliefs and practices about asessing sexual orientation in two veterans affairs hopitals. *LGBT Health* 1(3): 185–91.

Storey, J. D., Saffitz, G. B., and Rimon, J. G. 2008. Social marketing. In K. Glanz and B. K. Rimer, eds., *Health Behavior and Health Education: Theory, Research, and Practice*, 4th ed., 435–64. San Francisco: John Wiley and Sons.

Venere, K. September 9, 2014. *Let's Talk about Efficacy and Effectiveness*. Retrieved October 12, 2016, from Physiological: Where Physical Therapy Gets Logical: http://www.physiologicalpt.com/physiological/2014/09/09/efficacy-vs-effectiveness

Veniegas, R. C., Kao, U. H., and Rosales, R. 2009. Adapting HIV prevention evidence-based interventions in practice settings: An interview study. *Implementation Science* 4, article 76.

Wilson, C. K., West, L., Stepleman, L., Villarosa, M., Ange, B., Decker, M., and Waller, J. L. 2013. Attitudes toward LGBT patients among students in the health professions: Influence of demographics and discipline. *LGBT Health* 1(3): 204–11.

Wingood, G. M., and DiClemente, R. J. 2008. The ADAPT-ITT Model: A novel method of adapting evidence-based HIV interventions. *Journal of Acquired Immune Deficiency Syndromes* 47: S40–S46.

Beyrer, Chris, 24, 49
bias: participant bias, 95, 96, 256; response bias, 136–37, 163; sampling methodology and, 91; selection bias, 194, 256, 262, 265; test bias, 137; time-space sampling and, 200
Bickman, L., 262
biomedical interventions, 222–23
bisexual individuals: defined, 67; health disparities and, 39, 56–57; health research needs for, 50; intervention design and implementation for, 208, 272; LGBTQ-specific measurements and, 144; program development and, 245; sampling methodology and, 56–57; sexual health among, 41; substance use among, 61
Bowen, D., 210
Braveman, P. A., 8
Brazil: LGBTQ health activism in, 32; violence against transgender women in, 44
BRFSS (Behavioral Risk Factor Surveillance System), 57, 92
Bronfenbrenner, U., 149, 204
Bryant, L., 238
Bullough, V. L., 78
bullying, 117, 152, 214–15
Bye, L., 94

California Health Interview Survey, 92
California Quality of Life Survey, 92
capacity building, 238
CARE (Comprehensive AIDS Resources and Emergency) Act, 226
Carpenter, Edward, 66
Carter, L., 245
Catania, J., 94
CBOs (community-based organizations), 217
CBPR (community-based participatory research), 205–7, 217, 238, 246
CEDAW (Convention on the Elimination of All Forms of Discrimination against Women), 28–29
CEI (Corporate Equality Index), 132
Census data, 94
Center of Excellence for Transgender Health, 84

chain-referral sampling, 94–95
Charles, V., 282n6
church-based health interventions, 220–21
cisgender individuals: defined, 13, 62, 185; gender identity and, 71–72, 83–84; health disparities and, 7, 10; intervention development and, 208; LGBTQ-specific measurements and, 142; minority stress theory and, 109, 110–11; sexual orientation and, 187
citizen participation ladder, 238–39
clinic-based health interventions, 219–20
Clinton, Hillary, 31
CNU (Connect 'n Unite), 224
Coalition for African Lesbians, 38
Cochran, S. D., 92
co-design approaches, 270
cognitive dissonance, 164
co-learning, 238
Coleman, J. D., 221
collaborative partnerships, 240–41, 242–43
community-based health research and interventions, 45, 217–19, 272
community-based organizations (CBOs), 217
community-based participatory research (CBPR), 205–7, 217, 238, 246
community mapping, 209
community mechanisms of change, 226–27
community sampling, 93
Composite International Diagnostic Interviews Short Form, 92
Comprehensive AIDS Resources and Emergency (CARE) Act, 226
concealment of sexual identity, 150, 280
concurrent validity, 135
Connect 'n Unite (CNU), 224
Conron, Kerith, 61, 65, 184
construct validity, 133–35
content validity, 134–35
convenience sampling, 57, 93, 209
Convention on the Elimination of All Forms of Discrimination against Women (CEDAW), 28–29
convergent validity, 134

Logie, C. H., 139
Los Angeles Unified School District, 215
low- and middle-income countries:
    health activism in, 32; health
    disparities in, 39, 40, 41; intervention
    implementation in, 281; LGBTQ
    research in, 15, 17, 44, 49

Major Discrimination Scale, 20
Makutle, Thapelo, 33
Marshall, Z., 238
Martin, J. I., 191
Martinez, O., 224
masculinity: defining and measuring,
    77–78; gender expression and, 186;
    gender identity and, 71; sexual
    orientation and, 65, 77–78
Masters, William, 75–76
Matthews, A., 254
Maulsby, C., 282n6
Mayne, Xavier, 65–66, 68, 72–73
Mays, V. M., 92
McCall, L., 12
McMahon, J. M., 210
measurement, LGBTQ-specific, 129–48;
    adaptation of existing measures, 139;
    best practice considerations, 141–44;
    conceptual framework, 131–36;
    creation of new measures, 139–41;
    existing tools for use with LGBTQ
    individuals, 137–38; indexes, 131–32;
    items, 131–32; operationalization
    process, 131–36; reliability, 135–36;
    response bias, 136–37; scales, 131–33;
    social context impacting LGBTQ
    behaviors, attitudes, and norms,
    141–42; subpopulations within LGBTQ
    communities, 142–44; test bias, 137;
    theoretical framework, 130–31; threats
    to quality, 136–37; validity, 133–35
mechanisms of change, 222–28;
    behavioral interventions, 222–23;
    biomedical interventions, 222–23;
    combination interventions, 222–23;
    community, 226–27; couples interven-
    tions, 223–25; dyadic, 223–25;
    family interventions, 225; individual,
    222–23; patient-provider interven-
    tions, 223–25; policy-based, 227–28;

psychological empowerment, 226–27;
    small groups, 225; structural, 227–28;
    support groups, 225
Meezan, W., 191
mental health: minority stress theory
    and, 105–23; mood disorders, 153,
    154; research on, 41–42. See also
    depression
Mertens, D. M., 282n4
methodology: definitions, 61–90;
    Generations study, 118, 119–21t;
    importance of, 55–60; measurement
    issues, 129–48; multilevel approaches,
    149–58; sampling, 91–103; social-
    network approaches, 159–68;
    theory-based research, 104–28.
    See also definitions; measurement,
    LGBTQ-specific
Meyer, Ilan H., 93–94, 95, 104
Michigan Forward in Enhancing
    Research and Community Equity
    (MFierce), 246–48
Middle East, minority stress in, 43.
    See also specific countries
middle-income countries. See low- and
    middle-income countries
Miller, Robin Lin, 183, 253, 260
minorities, racial and ethnic. See ethnic
    minorities; racial minorities
minority stress theory, 105–23; concepts
    in, 108–11; health care service
    utilization and, 116, 117; intersections
    of gender and race/ethnicity, 115–16;
    merging with other theoretical
    approaches, 114–15; origins of,
    105–8; research on, 42–44, 111–18
Moll, Albert, 66
Molock, S., 221
Mongoche, Alim, 33
mood disorders, 153, 154
Morrow, G. R., 210
MPowerment Project, 271
MSM (men who have sex with men):
    church-based health interventions
    and, 221; community-based health
    interventions and, 218; drug use
    among, 42; health activism and, 32,
    34; HIV/AIDS research and, 5–6,
    40–41, 172; intervention design and,

MSM (*cont.*)
192, 193, 194, 225; LGBTQ-specific
measurements and, 139; recruitment
for research studies, 211; sampling
methodology and, 55, 94, 96; as
sexual minority group, 187; social-
network approaches and, 160–61,
162, 164–66; substance use and, 42;
use of term, 13
multilevel approaches, 149–58; general
psychosocial factors, 151; individual-
level factors, 150–51; LGBTQ-specific
factors, 150; structural-level factors,
151–56; structural stigma study,
153–56
Muñoz-Laboy, M., 224
Mustanski, B., 212
Mustian, K., 210

National Epidemiological Survey on
Alcohol and Related Conditions
(NESARC), 92, 153, 154
National Health and Nutrition Exami-
nation Study, 92
National Health and Social Life
Survey, 92
National Health Interview Survey
(NHIS), 73, 79, 92, 155
National Household Survey on Drug
Abuse, 92
National Institutes of Health (NIH),
112, 187, 271
National LGBT Health Education
Center, 268
National Survey of Family Growth, 92
National Survey of Sexual Health and
Behavior (NSSHB), 92, 93
National Survey on Transgender
Experiences of Discrimination in the
United States, 64, 84
Neal, J. W., 267
negotiated safety strategy, 171
neighborhood sampling, 93, 94
Nepal: criminalization of same-sex
relations in, 31; recognition of third
gender in, 38
NESARC (National Epidemiological
Survey on Alcohol and Related
Conditions), 92, 153, 154

NHIS (National Health Interview
Survey), 73, 79, 92, 155
Nigeria: anti-LGBTQ ideology in, 39,
280; criminalization of same-sex
relations in, 30, 34
NIH (National Institutes of Health),
112, 187, 271
Nkoli, Tseko Simon, 32
nominal scales, 132–33
nonbinary: research study recruitment
and, 209–10; use of term, 13
nonprobability sampling, 57, 93–94,
96–97
NSSHB (National Survey of Sexual
Health and Behavior), 92, 93

Obergefell v. Hodges (2015), 142
O'Farrell, T. J., 224
online ethnography, 96, 207
online health interventions, 212–13
online probability research panels,
92–93
online recruitment of research participants, 199
online sampling, 96–97, 165, 207
ordinal scales, 133
Outlaw, Angulique Y., 183, 260
OutRight Action International, 30
Out2Enroll, 227–28
Owens, Christopher, 91

Pachankis, J. E., 244
Pakistan, criminalization of same-sex
relations in, 30
participant bias, 95, 96, 256
participatory action research (PAR),
237–39, 256–57
partnerships for intervention program
development, 240–41, 242–43
Patient Protection and Affordable Care
Act of 2010, 227
patient-provider interventions,
223–25
Patton, M. Q., 282n3
peers: peer ethnographies, 206–7;
peer-referral sampling, 93; social-
network approaches, 159–68
Photovoice, 248, 249–50
physical violence, 42–44

place of worship-based health interventions, 220–21
Plato, 65
policy-based mechanisms of change, 227–28
Poppen, P. J., 221
Positive STEPS (Positive Strategies to Enhance Problem Solving), 219
post-exposure prophylaxis (PEP), 224–25
Poteat, Tonia, 37, 49
power mapping, 246–47
power sharing, 238
pragmatic trials, 263–65
predictive validity, 134
pre-exposure prophylaxis (PrEP), 223, 224–25
prejudice and minority stress theory, 107, 109
preventive interventions, 46, 48, 167, 174–75, 178, 283
privacy: data collection and, 85; intervention implementation and, 280; recruitment of research participants and, 211–12; reluctance to self-identify as LGBTQ and, 199; research ethics and, 191; right to, 29, 31
probability or population-based sampling, 91–93
program development for LGBTQ health interventions, 236–59; cultural tailoring of pre-packaged interventions, 253–55; focus groups for, 245; formative data collection, 244–45; in-depth interviews for, 245; intervention development, 251–55; literature review for, 243–44; participatory approaches, 237–40; partnerships required for, 240–41, 242–43; power mapping for, 246–47; social diagnosis in, 241–50
Project 10, 215
Project Muse, 238
Project VIDA, 241, 242–43
psychiatric epidemiology, 106
psychological empowerment, 226–27
psychosocial research, 41–42; case study, 42
Public Health Service (US), 108

quasi-experimental studies, 154, 228
queer: gender-queer individuals, 209–10; use of term, 13, 67
Queer Sex Ed (QSE) intervention, 212–13, 223

racial minorities: gendered racism and, 20; health disparities and, 9–10; intersectional approaches and, 211; intersectional stigma and, 18–20; LGBTQ-specific measures and, 143; social-network approaches and, 160–61
random-digit dialing (RDD), 94
ratio scales, 133
RDS. See respondent-driven sampling
recruitment for research studies, 194–200, 205–11; best practices and approaches, 205–7; couples recruitment, 195–96; for efficacy trials, 262; individual recruitment, 194–95; intervention effectiveness and implementation, 280; online recruitment, 199; participant bias and, 96, 256; recognizing diversity across LGBTQ populations, 207–8; research questions as basis for, 196–200; respondent-driven sampling and, 94–95; social-network approaches and, 165. See also sampling
Reich, S. M., 262
Reisen, C. A., 221
Reisner, Sari, 83
Research Design: Qualitative and Quantitative Approaches (Creswell), 141
resiliency: church-based health interventions and, 220; intervention implementation and, 273; LGBTQ-specific measurements and, 144; minority stress theory and, 110–11, 114–15, 117; multilevel approaches and, 151; research needs for, 44
respondent-driven sampling (RDS), 94–95, 97, 99, 209
response bias, 136–37, 163
Rhodes, S. D., 224
Riley, Erin, 184
Riordan, M., 282n6